Cochlear Implantation for Cochlear Nerve Deficiency

Yongxin Li
Editor

Cochlear Implantation for Cochlear Nerve Deficiency

Springer

Editor
Yongxin Li
Capital Medical University
Beijing Tongren Hospital
Beijing, China

ISBN 978-981-19-5891-5 ISBN 978-981-19-5892-2 (eBook)
https://doi.org/10.1007/978-981-19-5892-2

This Springer imprint is published by the registered company Springer Nature Singapore Pte Ltd.
The registered company address is: 152 Beach Road, #21-01/04 Gateway East, Singapore 189721, Singapore

Preface

Cochlear nerve deficiency (CND) is one of the most serious inner ear malformations, accounting for 2.5–21.2% of congenital sensorineural deafness and about 50% of single-sided deafness. There has been controversy over whether cochlear implantation (CI) is effective for CND. To date, with the enrichment of CI experience, increasing studies have found that patients with CND can benefit from CI surgery, but problems remain, such as difficulty choosing the implant side, bilateral implantation time, and postoperative outcomes vary. The Cochlear Implant Center at Beijing Tongren Hospital is one of the earliest centers to perform CI surgery in China. Based on the large population in China, more than 5,000 patients have been treated with CI surgery, among whom patients with inner ear malformations represent a large proportion. Research on CI of patients with CND is a highlight of our center. Currently, our center has regularly followed up with more than 300 patients with CND and conducted in-depth studies on preoperative hearing and imaging evaluation, surgical strategies, improvement and promotion of surgical techniques, long-term follow-up of postoperative outcomes, postoperative programming, electrophysiology test, and vestibular balance function of these patients. Relevant experiences and achievements will be introduced in this book.

Due to the particularity of embryonic development, patients with CND may be accompanied by various cochlear malformations. There are also particularities in radiology performance and auditory and electrophysiological monitoring of patients with CND, making it difficult to formulate a standard CI surgical criterion for CND. Furthermore, many surgeons have doubts about the outcome of postoperative results. The above problems limit the promotion and application of CI surgery for patients with CND, making many patients lose the opportunity to return to the sound world. Therefore, this book systematically introduced the embryonic development of CND, etiology, progress in radiology aspects, preoperative and intraoperative auditory and electrophysiological evaluation, surgical techniques, postoperative programming and outcomes, and vestibular and balance function. The implantation strategies of special cases combined with different inner ear malformations will be shown.

We hope that the book *Cochlear Implantation for Cochlear Nerve Deficiency* can help colleagues better understand the severe inner ear malformation and master routine diagnosis and treatment for patients with CND. We hope that by reading this book, more otologists can have confidence in CI surgery for patients with CND and thus benefit more patients.

Beijing, China Yongxin Li

Contents

The Embryology of the Cochlear Nerve and Its Radiological Relevance

1

Anandhan Dhanasingh

1.1 Introduction

The action potentials generated in the hair cells of the cochlea in response to external sound stimuli, are transferred by the cochlear nerve to the auditory cortex to be perceived as sound (Dhanasingh and Hochmair 2021a). The term "cochlear nerve" (CN) covers everything including the nerve bundle in the internal auditory canal (IAC), spiral ganglion cell bodies, and the peripheral nerve fibers that connect the hair cells to the organ of Corti (Waldman 2009). Congenital anatomical abnormalities at any level of the auditory pathway can result in some degree of hearing loss (Korver et al. 2017). In 2021, World Health Organization (WHO) reported that 5% of the world's population—or 430 million people—require rehabilitation to address a "disabling" hearing loss (WHO). The inner ear is associated with hearing loss in the majority of hearing loss cases and cochlear implants (CI) are currently the gold standard treatment option for conditions of sensorineural hearing loss (Dhanasingh and Hochmair 2021b). Similar to the phenomenon of natural hearing, the electrical stimulation from the CI electrode is picked up by the peripheral neural fibers connected to the neuronal cell bodies which are further connected to the cochlear nerve to reach the auditory cortex (Dhanasingh and Hochmair 2021c). While the cochlea is a well-studied part of the inner ear, the CN is still to be studied in detail from the point of embryology and its deficiency.

Cochlear nerve deficiency (CND) simply refers to the absence of the CN as visualized in the T2-weighted magnetic resonance image (MRI) or refers to a malformation characterized by stenosis of the bony cochlear nerve canal (BCNC) or internal auditory canal (IAC) (Glastonbury et al. 2002). The causes and the mechanism of CND are still unclear. While it is common sense thinking that CND could lead to a

A. Dhanasingh (✉)
MED-EL Medical Electronics GmbH, Innsbruck, Austria
e-mail: Anandhan.dhanasingh@medel.com

Y. Li (ed.), *Cochlear Implantation for Cochlear Nerve Deficiency*,
https://doi.org/10.1007/978-981-19-5892-2_1

loss of effectiveness from hearing aids and CIs, several studies have reported benefits of CI for CND patients in the presence of small, but not fully absent, CNs (Kutz et al. 2011; Mori et al. 2020).

Soft tissues including the nerves are better visualized in MRI than in the computer tomography (CT) images (Chang et al. 1987). With the advancement in MRI, it is now possible to visualize the nerve bundles in the IAC (Valvassori and Palacios 2000). A detailed pre-operative image analysis is needed to study the availability of the CN in subjects with congenital hearing loss.

This chapter aims to cover the embryology of the CN and its deficiency. Also, this chapter aims to capture the IAC of different anatomical types of inner ear with and without CND from MRI images. This is of particular significance to emerging clinicians in diagnosing and treating hearing loss with CI.

1.2 Embryology of the Cochlear Nerve

Embryology is the basis for understanding the structural integration in different organ system and is also the basis for understanding developmental disorders (Brown 2007). Since the CN is part of the inner ear, the embryology of the CN can only be studied in combination with the embryology of the inner ear.

The inner ear is a compound structure derived from tissues of neural crest, mesoderm, endoderm, and ectodermal origin, and includes the bones of the auditory bulla, nerves, blood vessels, and epithelial membranes carrying out various functions (Sawin and Morgan 1996). A pregnant woman's gestational period of 40 weeks is generally divided into 3 trimesters, each trimester lasting 12–13 weeks (Sawin and Morgan 1996). In the first trimester, the otic placode begins to form around the 3rd week of gestation. This is seen as a thickening of the epidermis (the outer layer of cells in an organ) on either side of the embryonic head (Fig. 1.1a) (Jackler et al. 1987). It invaginates (Fig. 1.1b) and separates from the ectoderm on the surface to form a spherical epithelial structure called otocyst (Fig. 1.1c). The ectoderm, which is the outer layer of the germ cells, transforms to several organs and glands, including the inner ear and the central nervous system through a cascade of genes. These genes are called proneural genes as they have the capacity to transform ectodermal cells into neurons. These genes belong to the growing family of basic helix-loop-helix genes (bHLH genes) (Fritzsch 2003). Around the 4th week of gestation, a group of cells (neuroblast) delaminates from the otocyst and migrate to be located between the developing inner ear and the hindbrain (Fig. 1.1d), which will later differentiate to cochlear vestibular nerve (CVN) inside the IAC (Warnecke and Giesemann 2021).

The formation of the primary neuron of the inner ear requires the vertebrate bHLH gene neurogenin 1, as described by Ma et al. (1998). The neuroblasts proliferate and differentiate to give rise to the ganglion cell bodies of both cochlea and vestibular portion of the inner ear (Cooper 1948; Altman and Bayer 1982; Moore and Linthicum 2007). This process is apparently mediated by the bHLH genes of the NeuroD family (Kim et al. 2001). From the 4th to 9th week of gestation, the

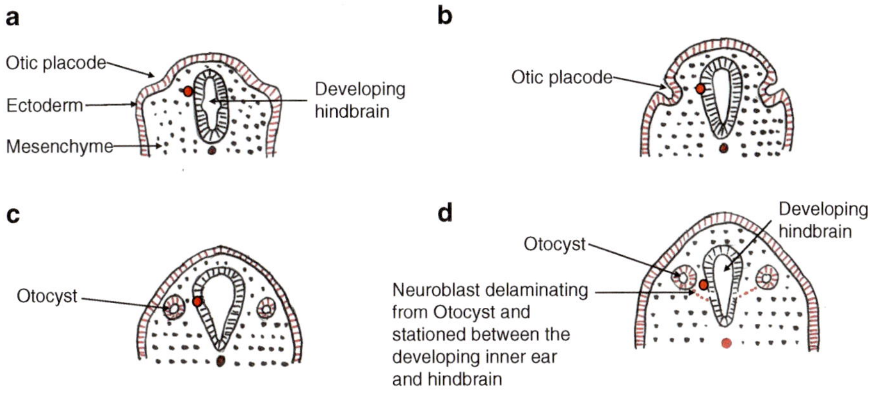

Fig. 1.1 Early stage of embryological development in the formation of inner ear structures. (**a**) Thickening of the epidermis marking the beginning of otic placode formation. (**b**) Otic placode further invaginates marking the beginning of otocyst formation. (**c**) Formed otocyst. (**d**) Neuroblast delaminating from the otocyst and migrating to be located between the developing inner ear and hindbrain

ganglion cells will develop towards the cochlea as well in the opposite direction towards the brainstem. Around the 9th week of gestation, the mesenchyme surrounding the otocyst starts to form the cartilaginous matrix which eventually ossifies and becomes the protective otic capsule. The cartilaginous matrix around the cells that are stationed between the otocyst and hindbrain, will eventually become the IAC. This process happens in parallel with the development of the CVN. Around the 10th to 12th week of gestation, the ganglion cells that develop towards the cochlea, form the base for synaptic connections to the developing hair cells in the organ of Corti, mainly in the basal turn of the cochlea (Pujol and Lavigne-Rebillard 1985). A similar pattern of ganglion cell growth towards the vestibular portion of the inner ear is expected. Brain derived "neurotrophic factor" released from the otocyst helps in the migration, growth, and the survival of the ganglion cells (Fritzsch et al. 1997).

In the second trimester, the peripheral neural fibers from the ganglion cell bodies form synaptic connections with the inner and outer hair cells of the cochlea extending from the base to the apex establishing the tonotopic frequency matching (Lavigne-Rebillard and Pujol 1988). During this time, the nerve grows in size and develops a more tightly packed cytoplasm around the multiplying axons. Schwann cells are responsible for the protection and the function of the nerve (Jessen et al. 2015). Around the 15th week of gestation, Schwann cells grow around the axons, which is the beginning of myelination (Fig. 1.2a). Around the 20th week of gestation, the axons grow to their maximum number and decrease to the adult level at the 22nd week of gestation (Pai 2017). In simple terms, a nerve is a bundle of axons transmitting electrical impulses. The myelination is a layer of insulation (Schwann cells) between the axons preventing cross-talk and enhancing the transmission of electrical impulses. By the 24th week of gestation, the myelin sheath is formed

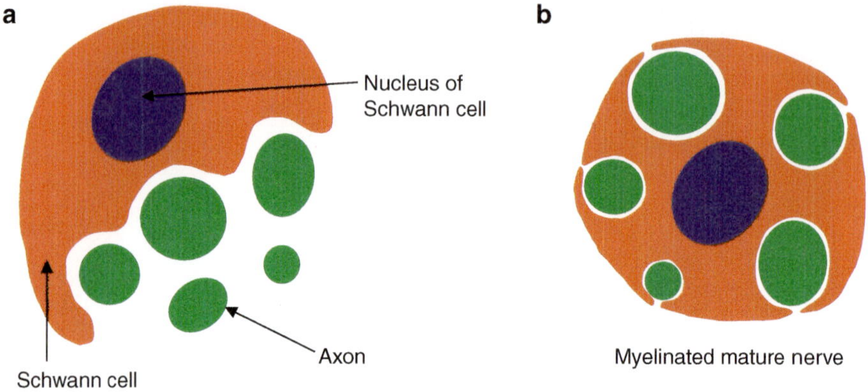

Fig. 1.2 Myelination of nerve fiber. (**a**) Schwann cell spreading over the axons. (**b**) Schwann cell completely covering the axons forming the myelinated mature nerve

throughout the length of the IAC, and it exits via the temporal bone (Fig. 1.2b) (Moore and Linthicum 2001).

During the third trimester, the CN and the central neural connections continue to develop both structurally and functionally and fetal responses to auditory stimuli have already started at this stage (Birnholz and Benacerraf 1983).

1.3 Cross-section of IAC of Normal Anatomy Inner Ear as Seen in MRI of a Pediatric Case

In a normal anatomy fully developed inner ear, the IAC carries one dedicated nerve bundle to the cochlear portion, two nerve bundles to the vestibular portion, and one nerve bundle to the face. This is clearly seen in the three-dimensionally segmented nerve bundles in the IAC as shown in Fig. 1.3a and in cross-section of the IAC at the mid-length between the cochlea and the end of the temporal bone as shown in cross-section-3 in Fig. 1.3c. As we go away from the mid-length more towards the end of temporal bone, the two nerve bundles of the vestibular portion merge to become one nerve bundle as shown in cross-section 2 of Fig. 1.3c. Just outside the temporal bone, the cochlear and the vestibular nerve (VN) bundles merge to form a single nerve bundle (CVN), whereas the facial nerve (FN) remains separated from the CVN as shown in cross-section 1 of Fig. 1.3c.

As we go closer to the cochlear portion, cross-section-4 of the IAC still shows four nerve bundles: the facial nerve, CN, superior vestibular nerve (SVN), and inferior vestibular nerve (IVN). The cross-section-5 through the cochlea shows two nerve bundles: the CN and FN.

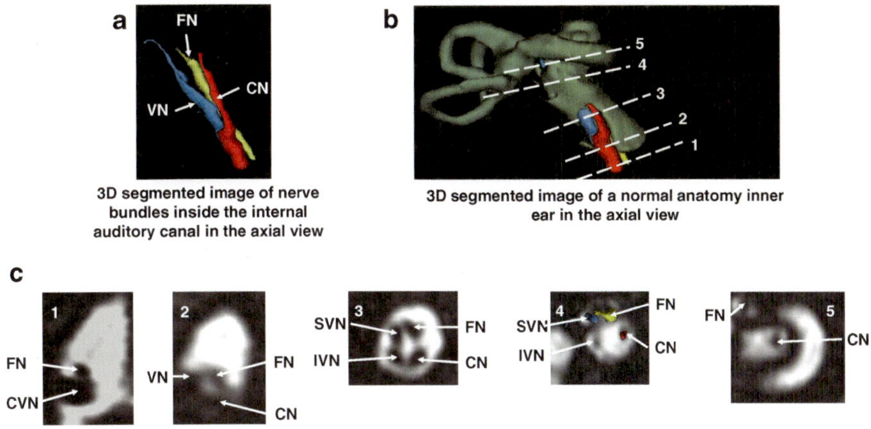

Fig. 1.3 Right side inner ear with normal anatomy of a pediatric case, showing the four nerve bundles. (**a**) The vestibular nerve (VN) is shown in blue, the facial nerve (FN) in yellow, and the cochlear nerve (CN) in red. (**b**) White dotted lines 1–5 show the cross-section of the internal auditory canal (IAC) at different positions. (**c**) Cross-section-1 is outside the IAC showing only two nerve bundles; one representing the FN and the other, the joined CN and VN to CVN. Cross-section-2 is just at the end of the IAC, showing the three nerve bundles of the FN, CN, and VN. Cross-section 3 is at the mid-length of the IAC, showing the four nerve bundles of the FN, CN, superior VN (SVN), and inferior VN (IVN). Cross-section-4 is close to the cochlea, showing the four nerve bundles of the FN, CN, SVN, and IFN. Cross-section-5 passes through the cochlea and shows the two nerve bundles of the CN and FN

1.4 Embryology of Cochlear Nerve Deficiency (CND)

As mentioned in the embryology of the cochlear nerve section above, the foundation for cochlear nerve formation starts as early at the 4th week of gestation with a group of neuroblast delaminating from the otocyst, positioned between the otocyst, and developing hindbrain. Any disturbance in the gene expression and cellular development at the 4th week of gestation that prevents the neuroblast delaminating from the otocyst could lead to the absence of cochlear nerve formation, so called "cochlear nerve aplasia" (CNA) (Lefebvre et al. 1990). Between the 4th and the 9th week of gestation, any disturbance to the ganglion cells developing towards the hindbrain and the mesenchyme forming cartilaginous matrix around the delaminating neuroblast lead to an overall inadequate formation of the CVN and the IAC as shown in Fig. 1.4b of a pediatric case, including IAC stenosis (Fig. 1.4c). Figure 1.4a shows the fully developed normal anatomy inner ear of a pediatric case with a clear connection between the IAC and the cochlear part and the VN branch indicated by the black arrow. However, the inner ear development from the otocyst may or may not be disturbed if the neuroblast has not delaminated from the otocyst which would result in the hypoplastic or absence of the IAC and the nerves.

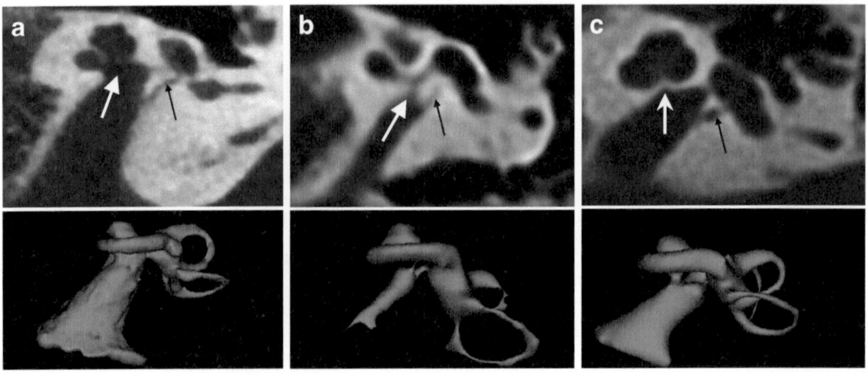

Fig. 1.4 Axial view of the fully developed inner ear by birth. White arrows point to the internal auditory canal (IAC) and the black arrows point to the vestibular nerve (VN) branch from the IAC to the vestibule. (**a**) Normal anatomy inner ear showing the IAC connection to the cochlear portion. (**b**) Hypoplastic IAC with a very thin connection to the cochlea. (**c**) IAC stenosis with the cochlea showing the VN branch connecting to the vestibule

1.5 Cross-section of IAC of Different Inner Ear Anatomical Types in Pediatric Cases

The brain derived neurotrophic factor (BDNF) that is released from the otocyst is the key for the development of cochlea, vestibule, semi-circular canals, endolymphatic sac as well the cochleovestibular ganglions (Fritzsch et al. 1999). Any disturbance to the pre-programmed release of the BDNF could cause deformity in any of the inner ear structures including the CVN. Figure 1.5 displays different types of cochlear anatomies as seen in pediatric cases, which is the result of developmental arrest at different time points of embryological development, however showing no disruption in the IAC. However, the two vestibular nerve (VN) bundles which are usually separated in the normal anatomy ear, appear as one stretched nerve bundle in the cross-section of the IAC in all the cochlear-vestibular malformation types other than the vestibular cavity type malformation. The vestibular cavity type malformation shows two nerve bundles in the cross-section of the IAC, the VN, and FN.

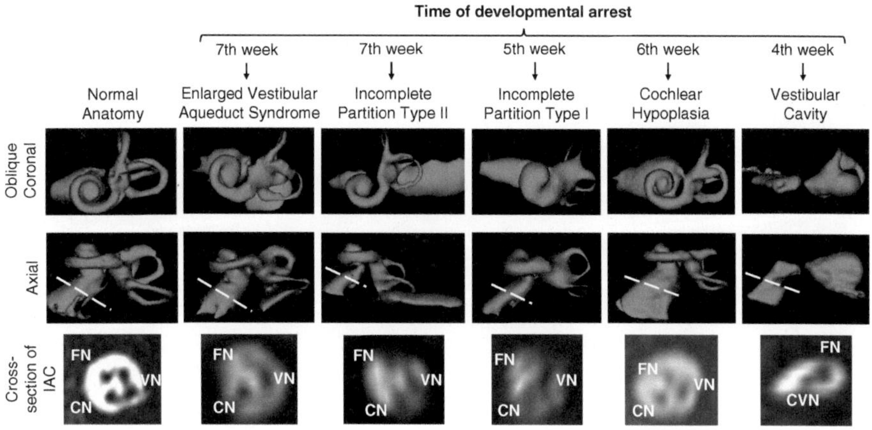

Fig. 1.5 Inner ear of different anatomical types shown in the oblique coronal view (first row), axial view (second row), and the cross-section at the mid-length of the internal auditory canal (IAC) (third row)

1.6 Cross-section of IAC of Different Anatomical Type with CND

In this section, pediatric cases with different inner ear anatomical types along with CND are presented and discussed. Figure 1.6 is a pediatric case with normal anatomy inner ear, but with an inadequately formed IAC bilaterally. The IAC is almost absent in this case.

Figure 1.7 is a case with cochlear hypoplasia along with CND bilaterally. The cochlear portion is developed for 1½ turns whereas the IAC appears very thin, and the cross-section shows no signs of any nerve bundle.

The absence of the nerve bundles in these two cases can be explained as the result of developmental arrest between the 4th and the 9th week of gestation that could have prevented the ganglion cells from developing/migrating towards the brain stem and the mesenchyme differentiating to cartilaginous matrix between the cochlear part and the brain stem.

It is known in the literature that the geometrical invariance known as symmetry is a prominent aspect of developmental morphology during embryogenesis. Pseudo-bilateral form of bilateral symmetry is seen in humans. However, developmental arrest often results in pseudo-random characteristics and minor stochastic deviations known as fluctuating asymmetry (Levin 2005). This could lead to asymmetricity between the ears with CND and inner ear malformation types. Figure 1.8 is a case with cochlear hypoplasia bilaterally. However, the IAC appears thinner on the right side with CN being absent, whereas the IAC appears normal on the left ear and shows the presence of CN. This can only be explained by the developmental arrest between the 4th and the 9th week of gestation on the right side with disturbed migration of ganglion cells from the otocyst towards the brainstem and no

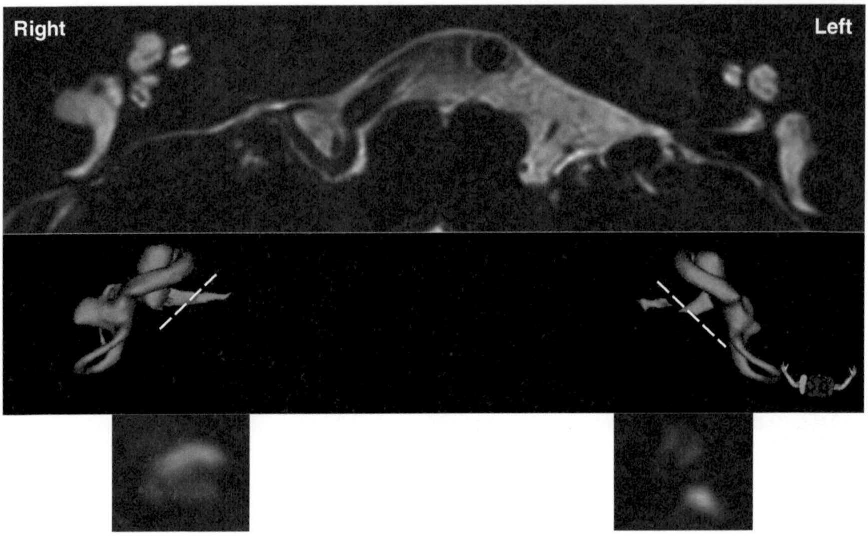

Fig. 1.6 Normal anatomy inner ear with an inadequately formed internal auditory canal (IAC) bilaterally. The cross-section of the IAC shows no nerve bundles indicating the cochlear nerve aplasia (CNA) or cochlear nerve deficiency (CND)

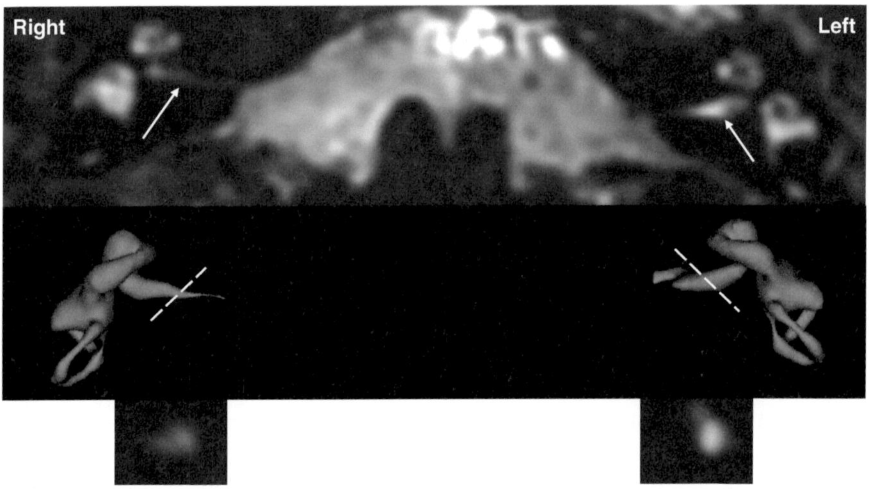

Fig. 1.7 Cochlear hypoplasia (CH) type malformation with an inadequately formed internal auditory canal (IAC) bilaterally as pointed by the white arrows. The cross-section of the IAC shows no nerve bundles indicating the cochlear nerve aplasia (CNA) or cochlear nerve deficiency (CND)

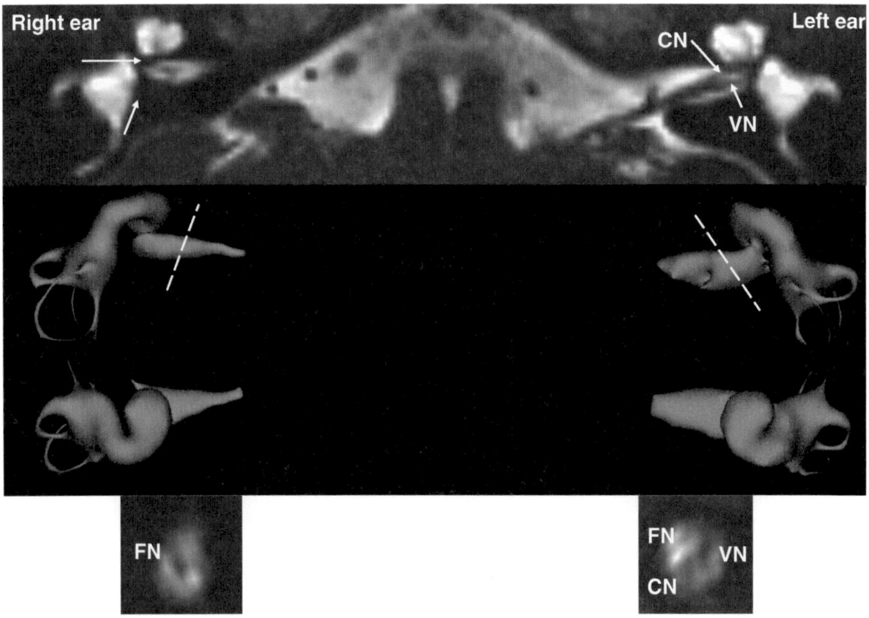

Fig. 1.8 Cochlear hypoplasia type malformation bilaterally with an inadequately formed IAC on the right side. The cross-section of the IAC shows one nerve bundle on the right side and three nerve bundles on the left side indicating FN, CN, and VN

mesenchyme differentiating to cartilaginous matrix which otherwise would have formed a normal sized IAC.

Figure 1.9 is a typical case showing different inner ear malformation types on either side. There is a vestibular cavity on the right-side and incomplete partition type-I on the left-side ear. The cross-section of the IAC on the right side shows two nerve bundles, one representing the facial and the other for the vestibular cavity. The cross-section of the IAC on the left side shows two nerve bundles, one for the vestibular portion and the other representing facial. However, the cochlear nerve bundle was not clear in the cross-sectional view on the left-side ear.

In extreme cases, the otocyst itself fails to form during the 3rd week of gestation and this condition is called Michel's dysplasia or also knows as complete absence of the inner ear as shown in Fig. 1.10 on the right-side ear. The left-side ear however shows the otocyst along with thin IAC indicating the arrested state of the otocyst between the 3rd and the 4th week of gestation.

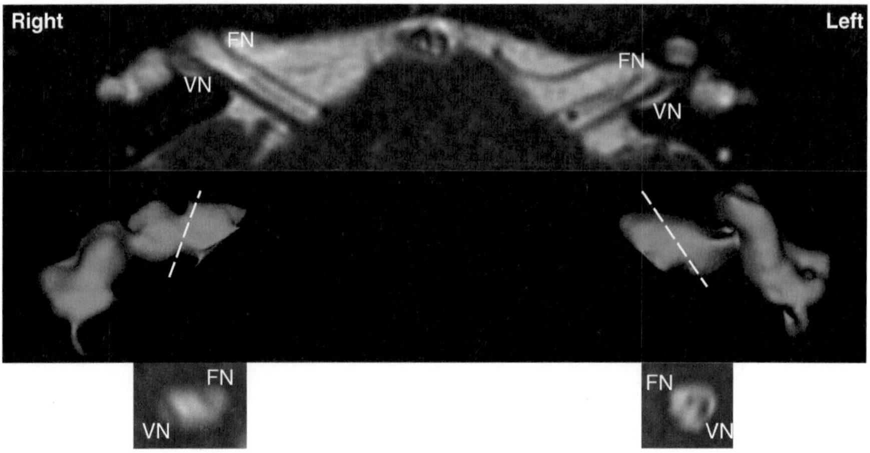

Fig. 1.9 Different malformation types on either side of the ear. Vestibular cavity on the right-side ear and the cross-section of the IAC showing VN and FN. Incomplete partition type-I on the left-side ear and the cross-section of the IAC showing VN and FN, but no clear CN

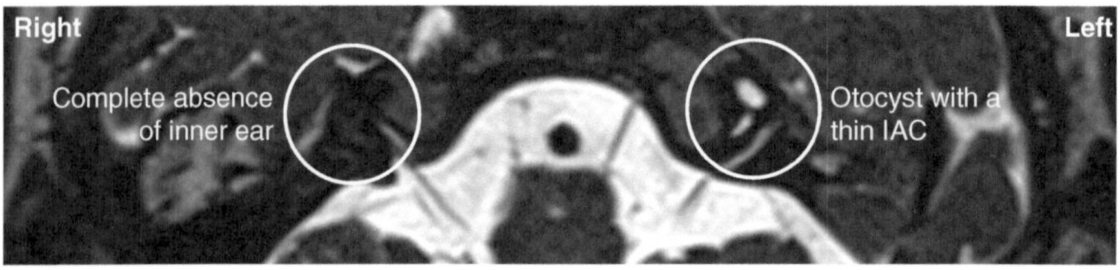

Fig. 1.10 Michel's dysplasia (absence of complete inner ear structures) on the right-side ear and a tiny otocyst on the left-side ear

1.7 Conclusion

The beginning of the development of the inner ear including the cochlear nerve starts at the 3rd week of gestation and ends close to the 12th week of gestation. Within this time period, the otocyst develops, releases neuroblast and neurotrophic factors which interact with each other throughout the whole development process. Any disturbance during this time period could lead to the developmental arrest of both the cochlear-vestibular part of the cochlea and the internal auditory canal carrying the nerve bundles. Identifying the cochlear nerve (CN) from the pre-operative image encourages the operating cochlear implant (CI) surgeon, because the CN is responsible for carrying the electrical impulses to the auditory cortex. A thorough knowledge of the embryology of inner ear anatomy and cochlear nerve development would help to relate the image findings and to push the research further into the future direction of gene and stem cell therapy.

Acknowledgments Dr. Una Doyle from MED-EL is acknowledged for language editing assistance and Mrs. Sea (Varachaya) Erhard, M.Sc. from MED-EL is acknowledged for 3D segmented image assistance.

References

Altman J, Bayer SA. Development of the cranial nerve ganglia and related nuclei in the rat. Adv Anat Embryol Cell Biol. 1982;74:1–90. https://doi.org/10.1007/978-3-642-68479-1. PMID: 7090875.

Birnholz JC, Benacerraf BR. The development of human fetal hearing. Science. 1983;222(4623):516–8. https://doi.org/10.1126/science.6623091. PMID: 6623091.

Brown MT. The potential of the human embryo. J Med Philos. 2007;32(6):619–33.

Chang AE, Matory YL, Dwyer AJ, Hill SC, Girton ME, Steinberg SM, Knop RH, Frank JA, Hyams D, Doppman JL, et al. Magnetic resonance imaging versus computed tomography in the evaluation of soft tissue tumors of the extremities. Ann Surg. 1987;205(4):340–8. https://doi.org/10.1097/00000658-198704000-00002. PMID: 3032120; PMCID: PMC1492735.

Cooper HR. The development of the human auditory pathway from the cochlear ganglion to the medial geniculate body. Acta Anat (Basel). 1948;5(1–2):99–122. https://doi.org/10.1159/000140320. PMID: 18876836.

Dhanasingh A, Hochmair I. EAS-combined electric and acoustic stimulation. Acta Otolaryngol. 2021a;141(Suppl 1):22–62. https://doi.org/10.1080/00016489.2021.1888477. PMID: 33818263.

Dhanasingh A, Hochmair I. Special electrodes for demanding cochlear conditions. Acta Otolaryngol. 2021b;141(Suppl 1):157–77. https://doi.org/10.1080/00016489.2021.1888506. PMID: 33818260.

Dhanasingh A, Hochmair I. Signal processing & audio processors. Acta Otolaryngol. 2021c;141(Suppl 1):106–34. https://doi.org/10.1080/00016489.2021.1888504. PMID: 33818264.

Fritzsch B. Development of inner ear afferent connections: forming primary neurons and connecting them to the developing sensory epithelia. Brain Res Bull. 2003;60(5–6):423–33. https://doi.org/10.1016/s0361-9230(03)00048-0. PMID: 12787865; PMCID: PMC3904733.

Fritzsch B, Silos-Santiago I, Bianchi LM, Fariñas I. The role of neurotrophic factors in regulating the development of inner ear innervation. Trends Neurosci. 1997;20(4):159–64. https://doi.org/10.1016/s0166-2236(96)01007-7. PMID: 9106356.

Fritzsch B, Pirvola U, Ylikoski J. Making and breaking the innervation of the ear: neurotrophic support during ear development and its clinical implications. Cell Tissue Res. 1999;295(3):369–82. https://doi.org/10.1007/s004410051244. PMID: 10022958.

Glastonbury CM, Davidson HC, Harnsberger HR, Butler J, Kertesz TR, Shelton C. Imaging findings of cochlear nerve deficiency. Am J Neuroradiol. 2002;23(4):635–43. PMID: 11950658; PMCID: PMC7975095.

Jackler RK, Luxford WM, House WF. Congenital malformations of the inner ear: a classification based on embryogenesis. Laryngoscope. 1987;97(3 Pt 2 Suppl 40):2–14.

Jessen KR, Mirsky R, Lloyd AC. Schwann cells: development and role in nerve repair. Cold Spring Harb Perspect Biol. 2015;7(7):a020487. https://doi.org/10.1101/cshperspect.a020487. PMID: 25957303; PMCID: PMC4484967.

Kim WY, Fritzsch B, Serls A, Bakel LA, Huang EJ, Reichardt LF, Barth DS, Lee JE. NeuroD-null mice are deaf due to a severe loss of the inner ear sensory neurons during development. Development. 2001;128(3):417–26. https://doi.org/10.1242/dev.128.3.417. PMID: 11152640; PMCID: PMC2710102.

Korver AM, Smith RJ, Van Camp G, Schleiss MR, Bitner-Glindzicz MA, Lustig LR, Usami SI, Boudewyns AN. Congenital hearing loss. Nat Rev Dis Primers. 2017;3:16094.

Kutz JW Jr, Lee KH, Isaacson B, Booth TN, Sweeney MH, Roland PS. Cochlear implantation in children with cochlear nerve absence or deficiency. Otol Neurotol. 2011;32(6):956–61. https://doi.org/10.1097/MAO.0b013e31821f473b. PMID: 21659925.

Lavigne-Rebillard M, Pujol R. Hair cell innervation in the fetal human cochlea. Acta Otolaryngol. 1988;105(5–6):398–402. https://doi.org/10.3109/00016488809119492. PMID: 3400441.

Lefebvre PP, Leprince P, Weber T, Rigo JM, Delree P, Moonen G. Neuronotrophic effect of developing otic vesicle on cochleo-vestibular neurons: evidence for nerve growth factor involvement. Brain Res. 1990;507(2):254–60. https://doi.org/10.1016/0006-8993(90)90279-k. PMID: 2337765.

Levin M. Left-right asymmetry in embryonic development: a comprehensive review. Mech Dev. 2005;122(1):3–25. https://doi.org/10.1016/j.mod.2004.08.006. Erratum in: Mech Dev 2005; 122(4):621. PMID: 15582774.

Ma Q, Chen Z, del Barco BI, de la Pompa JL, Anderson DJ. neurogenin1 is essential for the determination of neuronal precursors for proximal cranial sensory ganglia. Neuron. 1998;20(3):469–82. https://doi.org/10.1016/s0896-6273(00)80988-5. PMID: 9539122.

Moore JK, Linthicum FH Jr. Myelination of the human auditory nerve: different time courses for Schwann cell and glial myelin. Ann Otol Rhinol Laryngol. 2001;110(7 Pt 1):655–61. https://doi.org/10.1177/000348940111000711. PMID: 11465825.

Moore JK, Linthicum FH Jr. The human auditory system: a timeline of development. Int J Audiol. 2007;46(9):460–78. https://doi.org/10.1080/14992020701383019. PMID: 17828663.

Mori A, Kashio A, Akamatsu Y, Ogata E, Hoshi Y, Matsumoto Y, Iwasaki S, Yamasoba T. Long-term outcomes of cochlear implantation in children with cochlear nerve deficiency. Arch Clin Med Case Rep. 2020;4:990–1002.

Pai I. Embryology of cochlear nerve and its deficiency. In: Kaga K, editor. Cochlear implantation in children with inner ear malformation and cochlear nerve deficiency. Modern otology and neurotology. Berlin: Springer; 2017.

Pujol R, Lavigne-Rebillard M. Early stages of innervation and sensory cell differentiation in the human fetal organ of corti. Acta Otolaryngol Suppl. 1985;423:43–50. https://doi.org/10.3109/00016488509122911. PMID: 3864347.

Sawin SW, Morgan MA. Dating of pregnancy by trimesters: a review and reappraisal. Obstet Gynecol Surv. 1996;51(4):261–4. https://doi.org/10.1097/00006254-199604000-00023.

Valvassori GE, Palacios E. Magnetic resonance imaging of the internal auditory canal. Top Magn Reson Imaging. 2000;11(1):52–65. https://doi.org/10.1097/00002142-200002000-00007. PMID: 10782726.

Waldman DS. The vestibulocochlear nerve-cranial nerve VIII (Chapter 9). In: Waldman SD, editor. Pain review. Amsterdam: Elsevier; 2009. p. 22–5.

Warnecke A, Giesemann A. Embryology, malformations, and rare diseases of the cochlea. Laryngorhinootologie. 2021;100(S1):S1–S43. https://doi.org/10.1055/a-1349-3824. Epub 2021 Apr 30. PMID: 34352899; PMCID: PMC8354575.

Pathogenesis of Cochlear Nerve Deficiency

2

Lihui Huang, Cheng Wen, Jinge Xie, Yiding Yu, and Yue Li

2.1 Introduction

Cochlear nerve deficiency (CND) is defined as a thin or absent cochlear branch of the cranial nerve VIII, including the congenital partial or complete underdevelopment of the cochlear nerve and acquired degenerative changes due to various causes (Sha et al. 2014; Chinnadurai et al. 2016). CND is a postsynaptic lesion involving myelinated nerve axons and can be seen in children with normal cochlear outer hair cell function, so cochlear dysplasia is considered as one of the sites and causes of auditory neuropathy (Wang and Starr 2018). Currently, the etiology and pathogenesis of cochlear dysplasia are unclear and are generally thought to be related to congenital development and acquired degeneration (Wilkins et al. 2012).

2.2 Pathogenesis of Cochlear Nerve Deficiency

2.2.1 Congenital Development

CND includes unilateral and bilateral CND. Bilateral CND may result from an early developmental insult that affects both the hindbrain and cochlear formation, while unilateral CND might result from a later localized insult limited to the cochlear inner hair cells, spiral ganglion, or cochlear nerve itself (Huang et al. 2010).

L. Huang (✉) · C. Wen · J. Xie · Y. Yu · Y. Li
Department of Otolaryngology-Head and Neck Surgery, Beijing Tongren Hospital, Capital Medical University, Beijing Institute of Otolaryngology, Beijing, China

Key Laboratory of Otolaryngology-Head and Neck Surgery (Capital Medical University), Ministry of Education, Beijing, China
e-mail: huanglihui@ccmu.edu.cn

Y. Li (ed.), *Cochlear Implantation for Cochlear Nerve Deficiency*,
https://doi.org/10.1007/978-981-19-5892-2_2

More commonly, 40–85% of patients with CND have associated inner ear abnormalities (Carner et al. 2009; Adunka et al. 2006; Pagarkar et al. 2011). This association makes sense embryologically. The cochlear nerve develops concurrently with other vestibular and cochlear structures. Around the 4th week of gestation, the otic placode develops, it becomes the otic pit, and then becomes the otic vesicle. Around this time, ganglion cells form the acousticofacial ganglion, which later divides into the acoustic and facial ganglion. The acoustic ganglion divides into superior and inferior branches. The spiral ganglion, where the cochlear nerve neurons are found, develops from the inferior branch. At midterm, the cochlea achieves its final size and is surrounded by the bony capsule. The sensory epithelium continues differentiating, functioning around the 26th week of gestation. The soft tissues of the inner ear form after the bony labyrinth; the bony labyrinth may be normal with abnormal membranous labyrinth or other soft tissues. The development of the internal auditory canal (IAC) depends on normal caliber nerves within the canal to inhibit chondrogenesis, which is completed at the 24th week (Levi et al. 2013). Not surprisingly, there is a higher rate of cochlear malformations in bilateral CND compared with unilateral CND (Levi et al. 2013). Levi et al. assessed whether CND is associated with the brain or inner ear abnormalities in a cohort of children with auditory neuropathy spectrum disorder, and found that all patients with bilateral and 40% of patients with unilateral CND had associated inner ear malformations (Levi et al. 2013). Huang et al. noted an association between bilateral CND and labyrinthine and hindbrain abnormalities. Cochlear abnormalities were more common in patients with bilateral CND (73%) rather than those with unilateral CND (4.5%) (Huang et al. 2010). Zhao et al. also reported that unilateral cochlear nerve dysplasia can be associated with mild inner ear malformations, while bilateral cochlear nerve dysplasia is often associated with Modini-type cochlear dysplasia and vestibular semicircular canal malformations (Zhao et al. 2021).

There is a correlation between CND and the development of the IAC, and dysplasia or underdevelopment of the vestibulocochlear nerve is thought to be the cause of congenital IAC stenosis. Zhao et al. (2021) analyzed the relationship between CND and cochlear dysplasia and cochlear nerve canal dysplasia, and found that the degree of cochlear nerve dysplasia was closely related to the degree of cochlear nerve canal stenosis. The smaller the cochlear nerve canal was, the worse the cranial nerve development was, or loss was. There are two theories to explain the cause of IAC stenosis with cochlear vestibular nerve deficiency. One theory suggests that the stenosis is secondary to a hypoplastic vestibulocochlear nerve with the absence or deficiency of nerve growth chemokines, leaving the end organ absent and resulting in the inability of the nerve to grow and extend to the end organ; the other theory suggests that in the 9th week of gestation, the growth of the cartilaginous ear capsule is inhibited and eventually leads to the development of the primary bony ear capsule (Rubel and Fritzsch 2002). Glastonbury et al. (2002) proposed that the absence of all branches of the vestibulocochlear nerve results in hypoplasia of the IAC, whereas if only the cochlear nerve is absent, the IAC is moderately narrow. Acquired neurodevelopmental abnormalities may mean degenerative damage to the vestibulocochlear nerve caused by "injury," including vascular, traumatic, compression, or inflammatory injury, in the pontocerebellar horn region or in the IAC. If the vestibulocochlear nerve is hypoplastic or absent and the diameter of the IAC is normal, then a comprehensive auditory examination should be performed (Glastonbury et al. 2002). If the cochlear nerve is hypoplastic or absent, but the diameter of the IAC is normal, this should be considered in conjunction with the audiological findings.

2.2.2 Acquired Degeneration

The nerve typically degenerates following cochlear hair cell loss, and the amount of degeneration may considerably differ between the two ears and in patients with bilateral deafness. Vos et al. showed the first use of diffusion tensor MRI (DTI) to image the auditory nerve in five normal-hearing subjects and five patients with long-term profound single-sided sensorineural hearing loss (SNHL). Comparing DTI metrics from the deaf-sided nerves with that from the healthy-sided nerves in patients showed no significant differences (Vos et al. 2015). There was a small but significant reduction in fractional anisotropy in both auditory nerves in patients compared to the normal-hearing controls (Vos et al. 2015). These results are the first evidence of possible changes in the microstructure of the bilateral auditory nerves as a result of single-sided deafness.

There are a number of studies related to animal experiments on the acquired degenerative changes of the snail nerve, including animal models of SNHL and diabetes mellitus. The loss of cochlear hair cells in rats initiates degenerative changes within the primary auditory neurons of the cochlea. These degenerative changes include the loss of peripheral processes, demyelination, and ultimately cell death. This pathology will affect the biophysical processes involved in action potential generation and propagation to an electrical stimulus via a cochlear implant (Shepherd et al. 2004). The relationship between diabetes mellitus and the auditory/vestibular system has been investigated for more than a century. The primary pathological findings in animal diabetes mellitus model studies examining animals with "diabetes" are outer hair cells (OHC) loss with mostly preserved inner hair cells, pathological changes of the stria vascularis, reduced endocochlear potential, the battery that drives cochlea involving K^+ recycling with the stria vascularis, and changes in afferent auditory nerve fiber integrity (Elangovan and Spankovich 2019).

2.3 Cytomegalovirus and CND

2.3.1 Murine Cytomegalovirus

In the inner ear, the spiral ganglion neurons (SGN) serve the important function of conveying electric signals to the brain. Li et al. found that SGN apoptosis has an important relationship with SNHL induced by murine cytomegalovirus (MCMV), which is a persistent infection that lasts for at least 3 weeks in neonatal mice cochleae (Li et al. 2016). SGN apoptosis was related to the expression of Bcl-2 and Bax. Bcl-2 and Bax are the major apoptosis regulation genes in mammalian cells that both belong to the Bcl-2 family (Mohan et al. 2012; Li et al. 2013). Bcl-2 protein could inhibit apoptosis and prolong cell survival, whereas Bax could accelerate apoptosis through forming heterodimers with Bcl-2 as well as forming a homodimer with itself (Li et al. 2016). Numerous studies have shown that SNHL induced by MCMV infection is associated with a reduction in the number of SGN (Chen et al. 2011; Bradford et al. 2015; Sung et al. 2019). Chen et al. found that the SNHL induced by MCMV infection was not only associated with a reduction in the number of SGN, but also with the changes in the ultrastructure of the neurons (e.g., there is swelling of the endoplasmic reticula, ribosomes, and mitochondria) (Chen et al. 2011). The current studies have shown that the apoptosis, number reduction, and ultrastructural changes of SGN are important components of the mechanism of SNHL induced by MCMV infection in mice.

2.3.2 Human Congenital Cytomegalovirus

Fetal encephalon infection directly contributed to congenital CMV (cCMV) infection-induced neurodevelopmental problems by triggering neuroimmune reactions that harm nerve cells (Zhang and Fang 2019). These defects also came about as a result of CMV gene products inhibiting the proliferation and differentiation of brain progenitor cells (Zhang and Fang 2019). The cCMV infection can also prevent neural migration and synapse formation and indirectly cause placental inflammation, which impairs the fetus' ability to get enough oxygen. Early in pregnancy, cCMV can contaminate the fetal encephalon and impair neurodevelopment, leading to a variety of neurologic abnormalities, such as hearing loss, infections of the central nervous system, neurodevelopmental disorders, ophthalmic issues, cerebral neoplasms, infantile autism, epilepsy, and other neurological disorders (Zhang and Fang 2019). The auditory system may also be compromised by the cCMV infection. Children with hearing loss have been more prevalent over the past 50 years, and CMV infection is one of the leading non-genetic SNHL causes in developed nations (Stevens et al. 2013, Ciorba et al. 2009). According to reports, CND and CMV are the two most frequent causes of unilateral SNHL (Paul et al. 2017; Usamia et al. 2017). In our clinical work, there are patients with CND and cCMV infection, and we speculate that cCMV infection may be associated with CND, but the exact mechanism remains to be further explored.

2.4 Case Analysis

We have shared a case of CND with CMV infection below, along with our experience of diagnosing CND. A 10-month-old boy was referred following newborn hearing screening. After the hearing diagnosis, his left ear showed severe hearing loss and right ear showed normal hearing. His axial temporal bone CT scan showed that the left ear had cochlear nerve dysplasia and the right ear was normal. His mother tested positive for cytomegalovirus Immunoglobulin IgG with 118 U/mL during pregnancy. The infant showed cytomegalovirus Immunoglobulin IgG with 130 U/mL at the age of 10 months. We will conduct long-term follow-ups for the patient to observe the hearing in his right ear. This case indicates that CMV infection may be related to CND. In addition, we should pay attention to cCMV infection, especially in newborns.

2.5 Conclusion

The etiology and pathogenesis of CND are generally thought to be related to congenital development and acquired degeneration. Congenital developments include either early developmental insult that affects both the hindbrain and cochlear formation or later localized insult that is limited to the cochlear inner hair cells, spiral ganglion, or cochlear nerve itself. Acquired degeneration includes cochlear hair cell loss, and the amount of degeneration may considerably differ between the two ears. There is a correlation between CND and the development of the IAC. Furthermore, cCMV infection may be associated with CND, but the exact mechanism remains to be further explored.

References

Adunka OF, Roush PA, Teagle HF, Brown CJ, Zdanski CJ, Jewells V, Buchman CA. Internal auditory canal morphology in children with cochlear nerve deficiency. Otol Neurotol. 2006;27(6):793–801.

Bradford RD, Yoo YG, Golemac M, Pugel EP, Jonjic S, Britt WJ. Murine CMV-induced hearing loss is associated with inner ear inflammation and loss of spiral ganglia neurons. PLoS Pathog. 2015;11(4):e1004774.

Carner M, Colletti L, Shannon R, Cerini R, Barillari M, Mucelli RP, Colletti V. Imaging in 28 children with cochlear nerve aplasia. Acta Otolaryngol. 2009;129(4):458–61.

Chen J, Feng Y, Chen L, Liu H, Wang L, Wang X, Xiao J, Liu T, Yin Z, Chen S. Murine model for congenital CMV infection and hearing impairment. Virol J. 2011;8:70.

Chinnadurai V, Sreedhar CM, Khushu S. Assessment of cochlear nerve deficiency and its effect on normal maturation of auditory tract by diffusion kurtosis imaging and diffusion tensor imaging: a correlational approach. Magn Reson Imaging. 2016;34:1305.

Ciorba A, Bovo R, Trevisi P, Bianchini C, Arboretti R, Martini A. Rehabilitation and outcome of severe profound deafness in a group of 16 infants affected by congenital cytomegalovirus infection. Eur Arch Otorhinolaryngol. 2009;266(10):1539–46.

Elangovan S, Spankovich C. Diabetes and auditory-vestibular pathology. Semin Hear. 2019;40(4):292–9.

Glastonbury CM, Davidson HC, Harnsberger HR, Butler J, Kertesz TR, Shelton C. Imaging findings of cochlear nerve deficiency. Am J Neuroradiol. 2002;23(4):635–43.

Huang BY, Roche JP, Buchman CA, Castillo M. Brain stem and inner ear abnormalities in children with auditory neuropathy spectrum disorder and cochlear nerve deficiency. Am J Neuroradiol. 2010;31(10):1972–9.

Levi J, Ames J, Bacik K, Drake C, Morlet T, O'Reilly RC. Clinical characteristics of children with cochlear nerve dysplasias. Laryngoscope. 2013;123(3):752–6.

Li L, Wu W, Huang W, Hu G, Yuan W, Li W. NF-κB RNAi decreases the Bax/Bcl-2 ratio and inhibits TNF-α-induced apoptosis in human alveolar epithelial cells. Inflamm Res. 2013;62(4):387–97.

Li X, Shi X, Wang C, Niu H, Zeng L, Qiao Y. Cochlear spiral ganglion neuron apoptosis in neonatal mice with murine cytomegalovirus-induced sensorineural hearing loss. J Am Acad Audiol. 2016;27(4):345–53.

Mohan S, Abdelwahab SI, Kamalidehghan B, Syam S, May KS, Harmal NSM, Shafifiyaz N, Hadi AHA, Hashim NM, Rahmani M, Taha MME, Cheah SC, Zajmi A. Involvement of NF-κB and Bcl2/Bax signaling pathways in the apoptosis of MCF7 cells induced by a xanthone compound Pyranocycloartobiloxanthone A. Phytomedicine. 2012;19(11):1007–15.

Pagarkar W, Gunny R, Saunders DE, Yung W, Rajput K. The bony cochlear nerve canal in children with absent or hypoplastic cochlear nerves. Int J Pediatr Otorhinolaryngol. 2011;75(6):764–73.

Paul A, Marlin S, Parodi M, Rouillon I, Guerlain J, Pingault V, Couloigner V, Garabedian EN, Denoyelle F, Loundon N. Unilateral sensorineural hearing loss: medical context and etiology. Audiol Neurootol. 2017;22(2):83–8.

Rubel EW, Fritzsch B. Auditory system development: primary auditory neurons and their targets. Annu Rev Neurosci. 2002;25:51–101.

Sha Y, Luo DH, Li HG, Head and neck imaging. In: Otorhinolaryngology head and neck surgery, vol. 42. Beijing: People's Medical Publishing House; 2014.

Shepherd RK, Roberts LA, Paolini AG. Long-term sensorineural hearing loss induces functional changes in the rat auditory nerve. Eur J Neurosci. 2004;20(11):3131–40.

Stevens G, Flaxman S, Brunskill E, Mascarenhas M, Mathers CD, Finucane M. Global Burden of Disease Hearing Loss Expert Group Global and regional hearing impairment prevalence: an analysis of 42 studies in 29 countries. Eur J Public Health. 2013;23(1):146–52.

Sung CYW, Seleme MC, Payne S, Jonjic S, Hirose K, BrittW. Virus-induced cochlear inflammation in newborn mice alters auditory function. JCI Insight. 2019;4(17):e128878.

Usamia S, Kitoha R, Moteki H, Nishio SY, Kitano T, Kobayashi M, Shinagawa J, Yokota Y, Sugiyama K, Watanabe K. Etiology of single-sided deafness and asymmetrical hearing loss. Acta Otolaryngol. 2017;137(Suppl 565):S2–7.

Vos SB, Haakma W, Versnel H, Froeling M, Speleman L, Dik P, Viergever MA, Leemans A, Grolman W. Diffusion tensor imaging of the auditory nerve in patients with long-term single-sided deafness. Hear Res. 2015;323:1–8.

Wang QJ, Starr A. Hereditary auditory neuropathies: stepping into precision management from the discovery . Chin J Otorhinolaryngol Head Neck Surg 2018, 53:161.

Wilkins A, Prabhu SP, Huang L, Ogando PB, Kenna MA. Frequent association of cochlear nerve canal stenosis with pediatric sensorineural hearing loss. Arch Otolaryngol Head Neck Surg. 2012;138(4):383–8.

Zhang XY, Fang F. Congenital human cytomegalovirus infection and neurologic diseases in newborns. Chin Med J (Engl). 2019;132(17):2109–18.

Zhao JF, Zhao X, Zhang XA, Tao JH, Guo J. MRI manifestations of cochlear nerve dysplasia and concomitant abnormalities. J Clin Radiol. 2021;40(3):582–5.

The Value of Computed Tomography in Predicting Stenotic Bony Cochlear Nerve Canal

3

Bentao Yang

3.1 Introduction

The prevalence of congenital sensorineural hearing loss (SNHL) is approximately 1 in 2000 newborns and 6 in 1000 children by the age of 18 (Billings and Kenna 1999; Huang et al. 2012). SNHL may result from congenital or acquired abnormalities of the inner ear and/or cochlear nerve (CN). Cochlear nerve deficiency (CND) refers to the absence or decrease in width of the cochlear nerve and is found to account for SNHL in 12–18% of children (Parry et al. 2005; Mcclay et al. 2008). CND occurs more frequently in unilateral SNHL than in bilateral SNHL and is the most common type of malformation in unilateral congenital SNHL (Nakano et al. 2013). In children with SNHL, CND is usually a congenital deficiency, but it can occasionally be acquired after birth on account of degeneration of the CN (Glastonbury et al. 2002). In addition, children with CND may also demonstrate poor speech discrimination. The causes of CND are complex.

CND is a relatively common cause of profound SNHL that complicates the decision-making process regarding whether CI or ABI should be selected (Colletti et al. 2014). Therefore, it is of great practical importance for considering the operative approach. Hearing markedly improves in some children with CND fitted with CI, but they can't develop satisfactory speech understanding and production (Mcclay et al. 2008; Peng et al. 2017; Vesseur et al. 2018). Consequently, preoperative accurate imaging evaluation of CND plays a key role in selecting the optimal management strategy for these children. CND can be predicted on the basis of the width of

B. Yang (✉)
Department of Radiology, Beijing Tongren Hospital, Capital Medical University, Beijing, China
e-mail: cjr.yangbentao@vip.163.com

Y. Li (ed.), *Cochlear Implantation for Cochlear Nerve Deficiency*,
https://doi.org/10.1007/978-981-19-5892-2_3

the bony cochlear nerve canal (BCNC) by high-resolution computed tomography (HRCT) or cone beam computed tomography (CBCT).

3.2 The Prediction Function of BCNC for CND

BCNC is tiny canal that transmits the CN from the fundus of the internal auditory canal (IAC) to the cochlear modiolus, which can be clearly shown on both axial and coronal HRCT or CBCT (Fatterpekar et al. 2000; Glastonbury et al. 2002; Komatsubara et al. 2007; Clemmens et al. 2013). In routine clinical workup, the BCNC may be stenotic, which refers to the narrowing of the bony canal. In rare cases, when the BCNC cannot be completely exhibited by HRCT or CBCT, it is considered to be aplastic (Adunka et al. 2007). Previous studies have found that the severity of BCNC stenosis correlates with the degree of hearing loss. Moreover, there is a stronger correlation between BCNC stenosis and impaired speech discrimination (Purcell et al. 2015; Dong et al. 2016). Consequently, BCNC stenosis can serve as a reliable marker for CND. That is, when the BCNC is narrow, the CN is generally deficient. Although the BCNC stenosis displayed on computed tomography (CT) is a strong indicator of CND, magnetic resonance imaging (MRI) should also be performed for further clarification.

The cause of BCNC stenosis in children with SNHL is still unclear. Some investigators speculate that the absence or hypoplasia of the CN might affect BCNC development and thus induce its hypoplasia or aplasia during embryological development. Bilateral BCNC stenosis may be a result of an early developmental abnormality that also affects the brain and other neural structures, whereas unilateral BCNC stenosis may be attributed to a later developmental abnormality which is localized in the CN and cochlea (Casselman et al. 1997; Miyasaka et al. 2010; Clemmens et al. 2013).

Currently, BCNC stenosis belongs to a subtype of inner ear malformation, which is readily identified by HRCT or CBCT, usually accompanied with a short modiolus. BCNC is considered as a measurable indicator of CN anatomical or functional deficiency. Therefore, the measurement of the BCNC width may be valuable for predicting the CN status. Although standardized diagnostic criteria for BCNC stenosis have not been established, some authors have reported several criteria (BCNC width less than 1.2, 1.4, 1.5, 1.7, or 2.0 mm on axial HRCT) in the literature (Stjernholm and Muren 2002; Kono 2008; Teissier et al. 2010; Yan et al. 2013; Yi et al. 2013; Lim et al. 2018). In fact, the width of BCNC is easier to measure by CBCT, with more accurate results. To decrease the measuring error, the BCNC width should be measured at a special post-processed imaging workstation. Owing to its good diagnostic efficiency, we suggest that a BCNC width of <1.4 mm indicates BCNC hypoplasia, which may be highly correlated with CND. However, for children with unilateral profound SNHL, both BCNC and IAC simultaneously appear stenotic compared to the contralateral BCNC and IAC, which may definitely indicate CND with no need to further measure the width of BCNC. In children with some severe inner malformation, BCNC may be difficult to delineate by HRCT, thus there is no need to measure the width of BCNC as well. Komatsubara et al.

reported that patients with a narrow BCNC on CT were diagnosed as having CN hypoplasia on MRI with 88.9% sensitivity and 88.9% specificity (Komatsubara et al. 2007).

In children with SNHL, BCNC stenosis is generally associated with IAC stenosis, suggesting a strong correlation between these two entities. The relationship between BCNC and IAC stenosis is well established. The BCNC width seems to be a reliable marker of CN integrity in ears with IAC stenosis, while it seems to be an unreliable marker of CN integrity in ears with a normal IAC. That is to say, in ears with a small IAC, the narrow BCNC can help confirm the diagnosis of CND (Li et al. 2015).

The IAC is a bony canal that courses through the petrous bone between the cerebellopontine angle and labyrinth and transmits the facial and vestibulocochlear nerves. IAC stenosis comprises about 12% of congenital temporal bone anomalies, and it is usually unilateral. There may be variation in size of the IAC. The normal width of the IAC is approximately 4 mm and ranges from 2 to 8 mm on HRCT. An IAC with a width of less than 2 mm is defined as stenosis (Sennaroglu 2009; Masuda et al. 2013; Phelps et al. 2014). Although IAC stenosis is also highly correlated with CND, the correlation between IAC width and CND is not absolute. CND may occur in a normal-sized IAC, while a narrow IAC may not always indicate CND (Adunka et al. 2006). Thus, the IAC width alone may be insufficient to indicate CND, and combined stenotic BCNC may more accurately predict the CN status.

3.3 The Formation of BCNC

A narrow IAC with CND may be due to nutritional deficiencies before the 24th week of pregnancy, whereas a normal IAC with CND may suggest an acquired cause of SNHL. When patients have CND with a normal IAC, it can be speculated that an injury possibly occurred after the complete formation of the IAC, with only the CN getting injured, without any effect on the IAC size. The cause of acquired CND is more complex, it may result from the degeneration of the nerve fibers in the IAC after cochlear injury, in the form of either inflammatory, vascular, traumatic, or compressive injuries.

The vestibulocochlear nerve starts to develop during the 3rd week of pregnancy. During the 9th week of gestational development, the cartilaginous IAC is gradually formed together with the vestibulocochlear nerve. Some authors think that the IAC aplasia or stenosis may be owing to the absence of the vestibulocochlear nerve (Shelton et al. 1989; Macclay 2002). Thus, the presence of a narrow IAC on HRCT is often indicative of CND. The BCNC is also thought to be formed at this time and requires stimulation by the CN for normal development, which has been discussed above.

A BCNC width of less than 1.4 mm alone, an IAC width of less than 2 mm alone, or a combination of both, may be indicators of CND. The BCNC and IAC are complementary structures, and a joint assessment of both indicators should be performed by HRCT or CBCT to obtain a more accurate prediction of the CN status. However, MRI must ultimately be carried out for further verification (Tahir et al. 2017; Orzan et al. 2021).

3.4 The Value of BCNC

BCNC stenosis may exist in isolation or in association with other congenital inner ear malformations (Giesemann et al. 2012). Now we want to emphasize the isolated type, which means that the BCNC is narrow with a normal cochlea. Careful assessment of this type of anomaly by HRCT is crucial as it is frequently misdiagnosed in routine clinical work. While analyzing temporal bone CT images, an IAC abnormality may be more likely to attract our attention than a BCNC, which is why we must carefully observe BCNC in children with SNHL. In children with unilateral SNHL, BCNC stenosis can alternatively be identified by calculating the difference in measurement between normal and abnormal ears. In recent years, some authors have reported a high correlation between BCNC stenosis seen on HRCT and CND demonstrated on MRI, suggesting that CT may be a reasonable modality for CND identification in the workup of pediatric SNHL (Fatterpekar et al. 2000; Adunka et al. 2007; Wilkins et al. 2012).

BCNC stenosis is usually an isolated unilateral occurrence. It is considered as the most common anomaly in unilateral congenital SNHL. Bilateral occurrence may frequently be accompanied with other inner ear malformations. Although BCNC stenosis has a high prevalence in unilateral congenital SNHL, it is often underdiagnosed and unrecognized until early adolescence. Therefore, clinicians should not hesitate to closely investigate BCNC on CT as one of the possible causes of unilateral congenital SNHL.

BCNC stenosis can be found in some inner ear malformations, which are usually associated with a modiolus abnormality. Enlarged vestibular aqueduct, type 2 incomplete partition, type 3 incomplete partition, type 2 cochlear hypoplasia, type 4 cochlear hypoplasia, and isolated superior semicircular canal dysplasia generally have normal BCNC and thus their cochlear nerves are usually the thickest nerve in the IAC, which can be identified by MRI. However, complete labyrinthine aplasia (Michel deformity), rudimentary otocyst, cochlear aplasia, common cavity, type 1 incomplete partition, type 1 cochlear hypoplasia, and type 3 cochlear hypoplasia usually have a narrow BCNC, and thus their cochlear nerves are typically hypoplastic or aplastic (Sennaroğlu and Bajin 2017; Feraco et al. 2021).

BCNC stenosis appears to be a criterion for a negative outcome of the CI surgery, indicating that children with narrow BCNC may demonstrate poorer CI results than patients with normal BCNC. Chung et al. compared the post-CI speech performances among 3 groups of various BCNC widths (<1.4; 1.4–2.0; >2.0 mm). CND occurred more frequently in the group with a width of <1.4 mm, which also showed a worse post-CI outcome (Juyong et al. 2018).

3.5 CT Scanning Protocol of the Temporal Bone

The suggested CT scanning protocol of the temporal bone is as follows:

HRCT usually employs a multi-slice CT scanner (64 slices or more) in a helical mode, which can provide more fine anatomic details for the evaluation of the

BCNC. Currently, the procedure of temporal bone HRCT includes the raw image acquisition by CT scanning followed by image reformatted processing at an imaging workstation. The recommended protocol is as follows (HND of CCR 2017):

Scanning extent and image reconstruction algorithm: Axial scanning images are acquired (512 × 512 matrix) from the top of the petrous apex to the inferior tip of the mastoid. A bone algorithm mode is selected.

Scanning section thickness and plane: The raw axial images are obtained in a helical scanning mode with a section thickness of 0.5–0.625 mm, the thinnest slice of the CT equipment should preferably be chosen using the orbitomeatal line as the scanning baseline.

Reformatted section thickness and intersection distance, baseline and field of view (FOV): The acquired isotropic data of multi-slice CT can be used to perform multiplanar reformations (MPR). Both axial and coronal images are conventional reformations in routine clinical practice. The axial images are reformatted with ≤1 mm section thickness and ≤1 mm intersection distance, paralleling the lateral semicircular canal. Coronal images are reformatted with ≤1 mm section thickness and ≤1 mm intersection distance from the anterior margin of the petrous apex to the posterior margin of the mastoid, perpendicular to the lateral semicircular canal. Sagittal images can be reformatted whenever required. An FOV of 14 cm × 14 cm to 8 cm × 18 cm is selected on simultaneous bilateral temporal bone MPR and an FOV of 8 cm × 8 cm is selected on unilateral temporal bone MPR.

Window center and width: Images are shown at a window center of 500–700 HU and a window width of 3000–4000 HU.

3.6 The Comparison with Other Radiology Methods

Although HRCT is a traditional imaging modality used to assess the temporal bone at present, recent studies show that CBCT may provide better spatial resolution images and produce fewer artifacts at lower radiation doses compared with HRCT. Thus, CBCT has a significant advantage in assessing the pediatric SNHL and in delineating very fine anatomical structures such as the stapes (Kemp et al. 2020; Helal et al. 2021). CBCT can also show more excellent anatomical details of the BCNC and IAC compared to HRCT.

Although MRI is the most sensitive and precise technique for detecting CND, its scanning time is much longer and children need deep sedation during the scanning process. Thus, the initially diagnosis of CND is still based on CT findings (narrow BCNC, IAC, or both) and it is later further confirmed by using MRI. The BCNC and IAC are important indicators that need to be carefully observed in the assessment of temporal bone CT, especially for children with SNHL. We consider that children with both BCNC and IAC stenosis on HRCT, accompanied by ipsilateral severe or profound SNHL, are likely to be diagnosed with CND. In fact, the final diagnosis of CND must be proved by 3D high-resolution fluid-sensitive and heavily T2-weighted MRI (Shekdar et al. 2019; Quirk et al. 2019).

Although both CT and MRI play a fundamental role in the identification of ear malformation and CN status and further determination of the optimal treatment plan for children with SNHL, debate still exists regarding which imaging modality is better and should be the preferred choice for those children in routine clinical workup. CT has been usually regarded as the first line, but some authors argue that MRI should be the initial study of choice for those children (Parry et al. 2005; Simons et al. 2006; Adunka et al. 2007; Antonelli et al. 2010; Shah et al. 2018). We advocate an individualized approach in selecting the most appropriate imaging study for children with SNHL. The decision to employ CT or MRI should be based on the clinical history and presentation of the patient.

On the basis of previous studies and our experiences, the optimal imaging approach for a CI candidate is a combination of both CT and MRI. We recommend HRCT for the initial screening of all children with severe to profound SNHL. The width of the BCNC and IAC on HRCT can be estimated to further predict the CN status. In children scheduled for CI, MRI must also be performed in order to comprehensively assess the CN. Since the CN is less likely to be normal in the presence of isolated BCNC stenosis, auditory rehabilitation and language development after CI seem to be the most affected in children with undetermined CN status.

3.7 Conclusion

In conclusion, we would like to stress that an absent CN on MRI does not absolutely mean CN aplasia. It is likely that the CN is too thin to be detected by MRI owing to the limited spatial resolution of MRI, or it may occur within the facial or vestibular nerve fibers, and thus it cannot be identified (Thai-Van et al. 2000; Zdomu et al. 2010). In the future, this problem may be solved by using the ultra-high field MRI. Currently, those patients may select functional MRI or PET-CT study to further clarify the CN status prior to CI. In many CI centers, including our center, CIs currently continue to be offered to children with CND and those children are found to have hearing improvement, causing the speculation that some CN fibers are present but not visible by MRI. Therefore, the MRI diagnosis of undetected CN must be comprehensively analyzed in combination with the degree of hearing loss: (1) CN aplasia may present as total hearing loss or (2) CN hypoplasia may have residual hearing (Colletti et al. 2014; Li et al. 2015; Wei et al. 2017).

3.8 Cases Examples

Case 1. A 38-year-old girl with left chronic otitis media (Fig. 3.1).

Case 2. A 5-month-old girl with left SNHL (Fig. 3.2).

Case 3. A 6-year-old girl with bilateral SNHL (Fig. 3.3).

Case 4. A 4-year-old boy with left SNHL (Fig. 3.4).

Case 5. A 5-year-old boy with bilateral SNHL (Fig. 3.5).

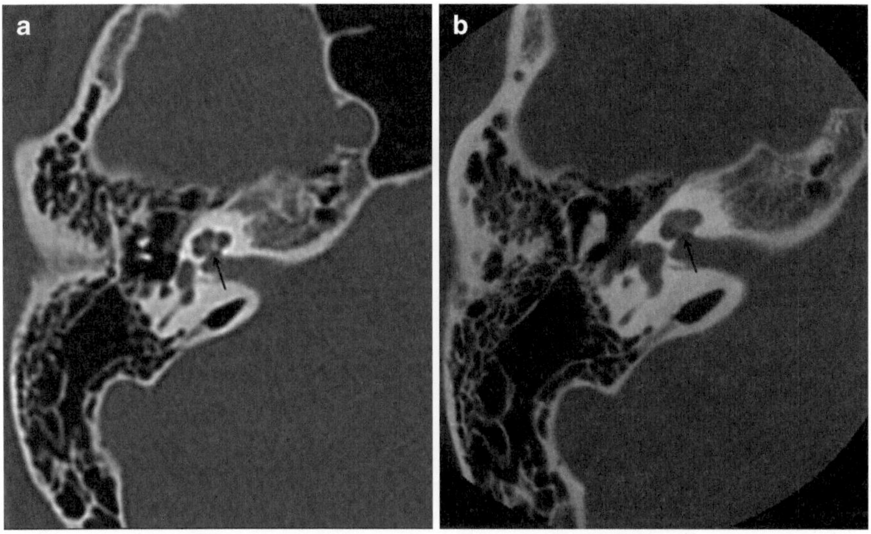

Fig. 3.1 Right normal bony cochlear nerve canal (BCNC) (black arrow) is seen on axial high-resolution computed tomography (HRCT) (**a**) and cone beam computed tomography (CBCT) (**b**). CBCT is superior to HRCT in delineating the BCNC

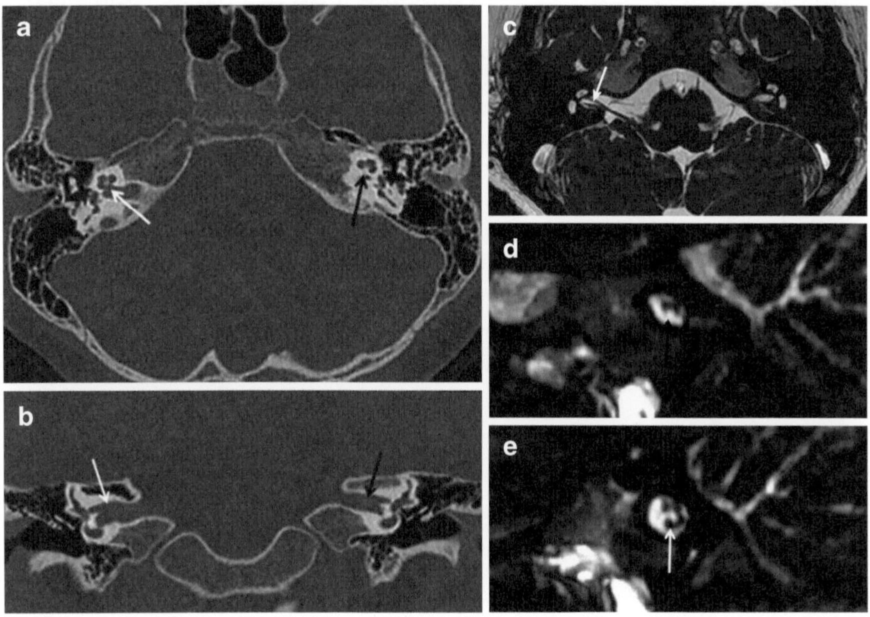

Fig. 3.2 The width of the left BCNC (black arrow) is narrower than that of the right BCNC (white arrow) on axial HRCT (**a**). Compared to the right IAC (white arrow), the left IAC (black arrow) appears stenotic on coronal HRCT (**b**). Axial 3D-FIESTA MR image demonstrates the absence of the right cochlear nerve (black arrow) (**c**). Reconstructed oblique sagittal MR images through the IAC visually demonstrate the absence of the left cochlear nerve (black arrow) (**d**) compared to the normal right cochlear nerve (white arrow) (**e**)

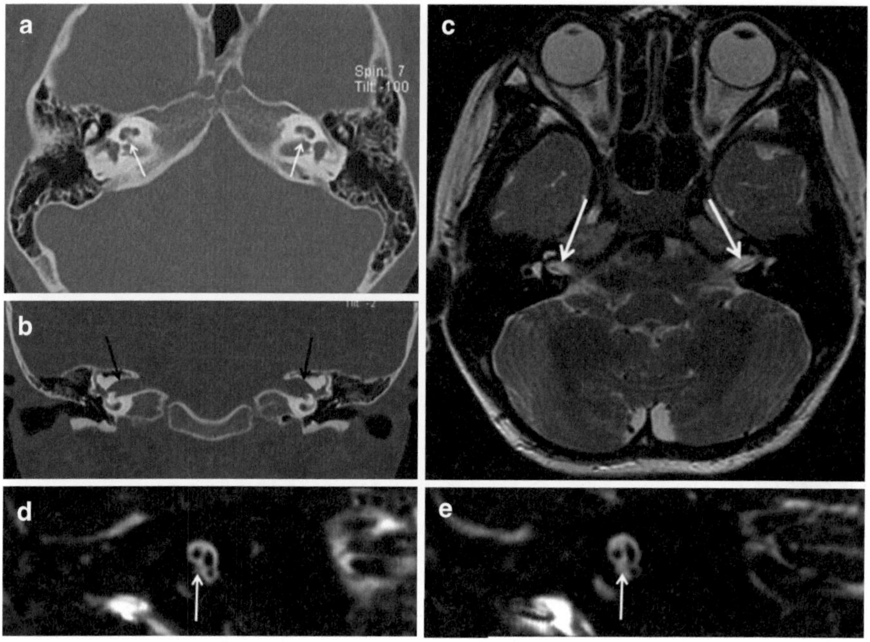

Fig. 3.3 Bilateral BCNCs appear stenotic on axial HRCT (white arrow) (**a**), while bilateral IACs have no stenosis (black arrow) (**b**). Axial 3D-FIESTA MR image demonstrates the absence of bilateral cochlear nerves (white arrow) (**c**). Reconstructed oblique sagittal MR images through the IAC visually demonstrate the absence of the bilateral cochlear nerves (white arrow) (**d**, **e**)

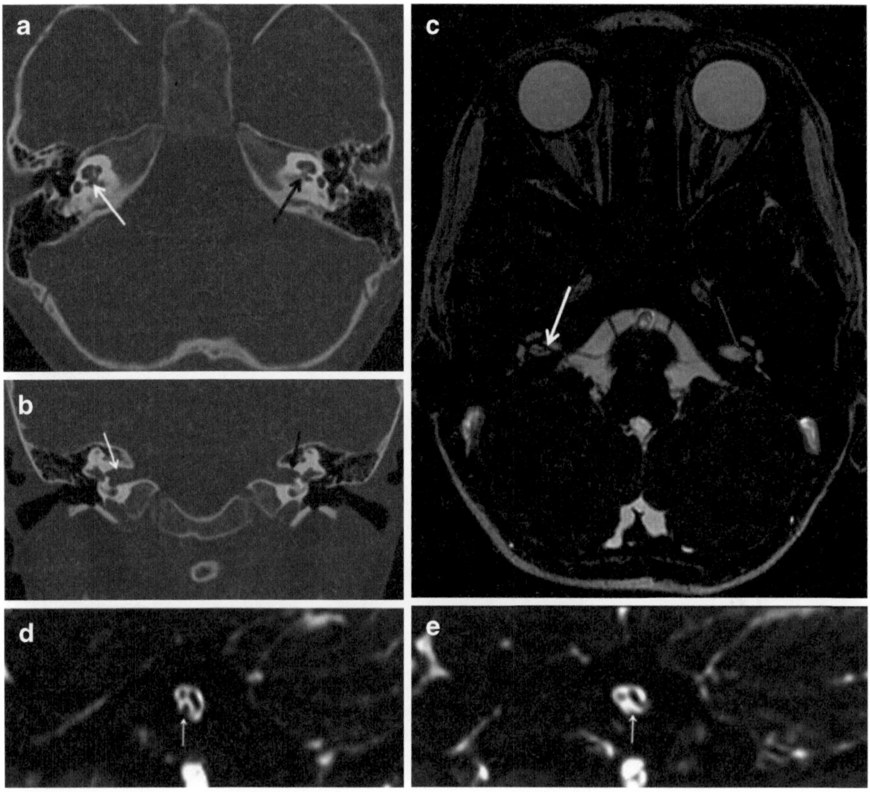

Fig. 3.4 The width of the left BCNC is narrower (black arrow) than that of the right BCNC (white arrow) on axial HRCT (**a**), while bilateral IACs appear symmetric with no stenosis (**b**). The left fine cochlear nerve is identified on axial 3D-FIESTA MR image (red arrow) (**c**). Reconstructed oblique sagittal MR images through the IAC visually demonstrate the right normal cochlear nerve (white arrow) (**d**) compared to the left tiny cochlear nerve (white arrow) (**e**)

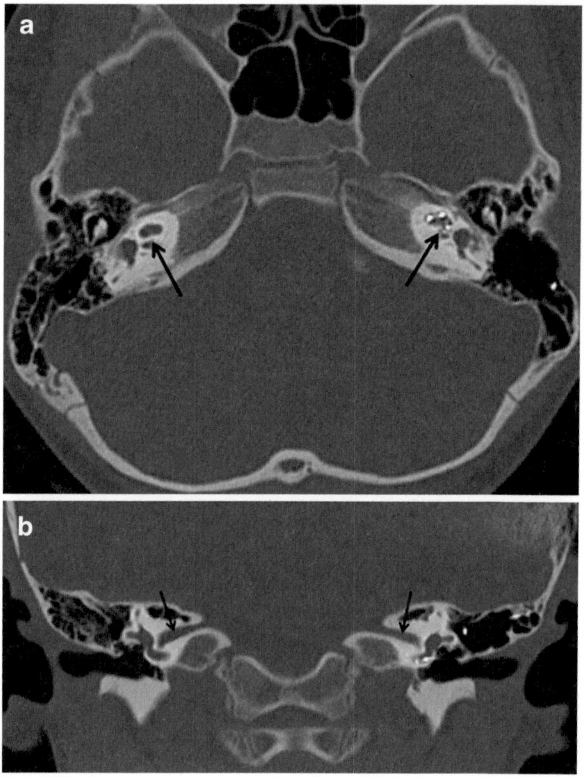

Fig. 3.5 Bilateral BCNCs and IACs appear stenotic on both axial and coronal HRCT (black arrow) (**a**, **b**). CI was performed on the left ear

References

Adunka OF, Roush PA, et al. Internal Auditory Canal morphology in children with cochlear nerve deficiency. Otol Neurotol. 2006;27(6):793–801.

Adunka OF, Jewells V, et al. Value of computed tomography in the evaluation of children with cochlear nerve deficiency. Otol Neurotol. 2007;28(5):597–604.

Antonelli PJ, Varela AE, et al. Diagnostic yield of high-resolution computed tomography for pediatric sensorineural hearing loss. Laryngoscope. 2010;109(10):1642–7.

Billings KR, Kenna MA. Causes of pediatric sensorineural hearing loss: yesterday and today. Arch Otolaryngol Head Neck Surg. 1999;125(5):517–21.

Casselman JW, Offeciers FE, et al. Aplasia and hypoplasia of the vestibulocochlear nerve: diagnosis with MR imaging. Radiology. 1997;202(3):773.

Clemmens CS, Guidi J, et al. Unilateral cochlear nerve deficiency in children. Otolaryngol Head Neck Surg. 2013;149(2):318–25.

Colletti L, et al. The therapeutic dilemma of cochlear nerve deficiency: cochlear or brainstem implantation? Otolaryngol Head Neck Surg. 2014;151(2):308–14.

Dong HK, Lee MJ, et al. Prediction of cochlear implant outcomes in patients with prelingual deafness. Clin Exp Otorhinolaryngol. 2016;9(3):220–5.

Fatterpekar GM, Mukherji SK, et al. Hypoplasia of the bony canal for the cochlear nerve in patients with congenital sensorineural hearing loss: initial observations. Radiology. 2000;215(1):243–6.

Feraco P, Piccinini S, et al. Imaging of inner ear malformations: a primer for radiologists. Radiol Med. 2021;126(10):1282–95.

Giesemann AM, Kontorinis G, et al. The vestibulocochlear nerve: aplasia and hypoplasia in combination with inner ear malformations. Eur Radiol. 2012;22(3):519–24.

Glastonbury CM, Davidson HC, et al. Imaging findings of cochlear nerve deficiency. Am J Neuroradiol. 2002;23(4):635–43.

Helal RA, Jacob R, et al. Cone-beam CT versus multidetector CT in postoperative cochlear implant imaging: evaluation of image quality and radiation dose. Am J Neuroradiol. 2021;42(2):362–7.

HND of CCR. Ear CT and MRI examination and diagnosis expert consensus. Chin J Radiol. 2017;9(51):654–9.

Huang BY, Zdanski C, et al. Pediatric sensorineural hearing loss, part 2: syndromic and acquired causes. Am J Neuroradiol. 2012;33(3):399–406.

Juyong C, Hun JJ, et al. Does the width of the bony cochlear nerve canal predict the outcomes of cochlear implantation? Biomed Res Int. 2018;2018:5675848.

Kemp P, Stralen JV, et al. Cone-beam CT compared to multi-slice CT for the diagnostic analysis of conductive hearing loss: a feasibility study. J Int Adv Otol. 2020;16(2):222–6.

Komatsubara S, Haruta A, et al. Evaluation of cochlear nerve imaging in severe congenital sensorineural hearing loss. ORL. 2007;69(3):198–202.

Kono T. Computed tomographic features of the bony canal of the cochlear nerve in pediatric patients with unilateral sensorineural hearing loss. Radiat Med. 2008;26(3):115.

Li Y, Yang J, et al. Restudy of malformations of the internal auditory meatus, cochlear nerve canal and cochlear nerve. Eur Arch Otorhinolaryngol. 2015;272(7):1587–96.

Lim CAH, Lim JH, et al. Bony cochlear nerve canal stenosis in pediatric unilateral sensorineural hearing loss. Int J Pediatr Otorhinolaryngol. 2018;106:72–4.

Macclay J. Major and minor temporal bone abnormalities in children with and without congenital sensorineural hearing loss. Arch Otolaryngol Head Neck Surg. 2002;128(6):664–71.

Masuda S, Usui S, et al. High prevalence of inner-ear and/or internal auditory canal malformations in children with unilateral sensorineural hearing loss. Int J Pediatr Otorhinolaryngol. 2013;77(2):228–32.

Mcclay JE, Booth TN, et al. Evaluation of pediatric sensorineural hearing loss with magnetic resonance imaging. Arch Otolaryngol Head Neck Surg. 2008;134(9):945.

Miyasaka M, Nosaka S, et al. CT and MR imaging for pediatric cochlear implantation: emphasis on the relationship between the cochlear nerve canal and the cochlear nerve. Pediatr Radiol. 2010;40(9):1509–16.

Nakano A, Arimoto Y, et al. Cochlear nerve deficiency and associated clinical features in patients with bilateral and unilateral hearing loss. Otol Neurotol. 2013;34(3):554–8.

Orzan E, Pizzamiglio G, et al. Correlation of cochlear aperture stenosis with cochlear nerve deficiency in congenital unilateral hearing loss and prognostic relevance for cochlear implantation. Sci Rep. 2021;1(11):3338.

Parry DA, Booth T, et al. Advantages of magnetic resonance imaging over computed tomography in preoperative evaluation of pediatric cochlear implant candidates. Otol Neurotol. 2005;26(5):976–82.

Peng KA, Kuan EC, et al. Cochlear nerve aplasia and hypoplasia: predictors of cochlear implant success. Otolaryngol Head Neck Surg. 2017;157(3):194599817718798.

Phelps PD, Annis J, et al. Imaging for cochlear implants. Br J Radiol. 2014;63(751):512–6.

Purcell PL, Iwata AJ, et al. Bony cochlear nerve canal stenosis and speech discrimination in pediatric unilateral hearing loss. Laryngoscope. 2015;125(7):1691–6.

Quirk B, Youssef A, et al. Radiological diagnosis of the inner ear malformations in children with sensorineural hearing loss. BJR Open. 2019;1(1):20180050.

Sennaroglu L. Cochlear implantation in inner ear malformations—a review article. Cochlear Implants Int. 2009;11(1):4–41.

Sennaroğlu L, Bajin MD. Classification and current management of inner ear malformations. Balkan Med J. 2017;34(5):397–411.

Shah J, et al. Evaluating diagnostic yield of computed tomography (CT) and magnetic resonance imaging (MRI) in pediatric unilateral sensorineural hearing loss. Int J Pediatr Otorhinolaryngol. 2018;115:41–4.

Shekdar KV, et al. Imaging of pediatric hearing loss. Neuroimaging Clin N Am. 2019;29(1):103–15.

Shelton C, Luxford WM, et al. The narrow internal Auditory Canal in children: a contraindication to cochlear implants. Otolaryngol Head Neck Surg. 1989;100(3):227–31.

Simons JP, Mandell DL, et al. Computed tomography and magnetic resonance imaging in pediatric unilateral and asymmetric sensorineural hearing loss. Arch Otolaryngol Head Neck Surg. 2006;132(2):186–92.

Stjernholm C, Muren C. Dimensions of the cochlear nerve canal: a radioanatomic investigation. Acta Otolaryngol. 2002;122(1):43–8.

Tahir E, Bajin MD, et al. Bony cochlear nerve canal and internal auditory canal measures predict cochlear nerve status. J Laryngol Otol. 2017;131(8):676–83.

Teissier N, Abbeele T, et al. Computed tomography measurements of the normal and the pathologic cochlea in children. Pediatr Radiol. 2010;40(3):275–83.

Thai-Van H, Fraysse B, et al. Functional magnetic resonance imaging may avoid misdiagnosis of cochleovestibular nerve aplasia in congenital deafness. Otol Neurotol. 2000;21(5):663.

Vesseur A, Free R, et al. Hearing restoration in cochlear nerve deficiency: the choice between cochlear implant or auditory brainstem implant, a meta-analysis. Otol Neurotol. 2018;39(4):428–37.

Wei X, Li Y, et al. Predicting auditory outcomes from radiological imaging in cochlear implant patients with cochlear nerve deficiency. Otol Neurotol. 2017;38(5):685–93.

Wilkins A, Prabhu SP, et al. Frequent association of cochlear nerve canal stenosis with pediatric sensorineural hearing loss. Arch Otolaryngol Head Neck Surg. 2012;138(4):383–8.

Yan F, Li J, et al. The cochlear nerve canal and internal auditory canal in children with normal cochlea but cochlear nerve deficiency. Acta Radiol. 2013;54(3):292–8.

Yi JS, Lim HW, et al. Proportion of bony cochlear nerve canal anomalies in unilateral sensorineural hearing loss in children. Int J Pediatr Otorhinolaryngol. 2013;77(4):530–3.

Zdomu M, Sezen O, et al. Connections between the facial, vestibular and cochlear nerve bundles within the internal auditory canal. J Anat. 2010;205(1):65–75.

4 Magnetic Resonance Imaging Evaluation of Cochlear Nerve Deficiency

Jianhong Li and Junfang Xian

4.1 Introduction

Cochlear nerve deficiency (CND) is a relatively common cause of congenital sensorineural hearing loss (SNHL) and includes cochlear nerve aplasia and hypoplasia. The size or presence of the cochlear nerve could be evaluated using T2-weighted MR imaging with oblique parasagittal fast spin-echo (Rubinstein et al. 1996). Subsequently, a more detailed evaluation of nerves in the internal auditory canal (IAC) was made possible using highly contrasted T2-weighted images. In most cases, the size of the cochlear nerve was reported to be similar to or slightly larger than that of the facial nerve (FN) (Kim et al. 1998). However, in cases where the cochlear nerve is significantly smaller than the FN in IAC, it is considered cochlear nerve hypoplasia. Cochlear nerve aplasia is the absence of a cochlear nerve within the IAC (Casselman et al. 1997).

CND accounts for 12–18% of children with SNHL (Parry et al. 2005; Mcclay et al. 2008). CND occurs more frequently in unilateral SNHL than in bilateral SNHL (Nakano et al. 2013); CDN was found in approximately 25–48% of patients with unilateral hearing loss (Clemmens et al. 2013; Usami et al. 2017; Lin et al. 2017) and 15.4% of patients with severe-to-profound bilateral hearing loss (Dagkiran et al. 2016). The causes of CND are complex; it may have been due to congenital hypoplasia of the nerve or acquired degeneration or atrophy (Glastonbury et al. 2002).

Children with CND who receive a cochlear implant (CI) generally exhibit poorer auditory performance than children with CI without CND. In contrast, many recent studies reported that some children with CND fitted with CI had improved hearing

J. Li · J. Xian (✉)
Department of Radiology, Beijing Tongren Hospital, Capital Medical University, Beijing, China
e-mail: cjr.xianjunfang@vip.163.com

Y. Li (ed.), *Cochlear Implantation for Cochlear Nerve Deficiency*,
https://doi.org/10.1007/978-981-19-5892-2_4

but could not develop satisfactory speech understanding and production (Mcclay et al. 2008; Peng et al. 2017; Vesseur et al. 2018). CND perplexes the decision-making process regarding the selection of CI or auditory brainstem implant (ABI) (Liliana et al. 2014). Therefore, it is of great practical importance for operative consideration before CI. Consequently, a precise preoperative magnetic resonance imaging (MRI) evaluation of CND plays a key role in selecting the optimal management strategy for these children. However, there are some limitations to MRI as a diagnostic approach for CND. Preoperative evaluation of CI requires comprehensive consideration of imaging and clinical factors.

4.2 MRI Findings of CND

MRI can be used to recognize the course and distribution of inner ear and cisternal segments of vestibular cochlear nerve (VCN). High-resolution 3D MRI at 3.0 T has been widely used to display the vestibular cochlear nerve (Held et al. 1997; Lane et al. 2004; Herman and Angeli 2011). Using high signal intensity, high signal-to-noise ratio, and high contrast resolution, an oblique sagittal MR image was used to describe the neuromorphology in the IAC. In the oblique sagittal plane imaging, the FN and the three divisions of the vestibulocochlear nerve (superior vestibular, inferior vestibular, and cochlear nerve) can be easily identified in the distal or middle part of the IAC in normal subjects (Fig. 4.1). The FN lies in the anterosuperior portion, the cochlear nerve lies in the anteroinferior portion, and the superior and inferior vestibular nerves lie in the posterior portion of the canal (Rubinstein et al. 1996; Kim et al. 1998).

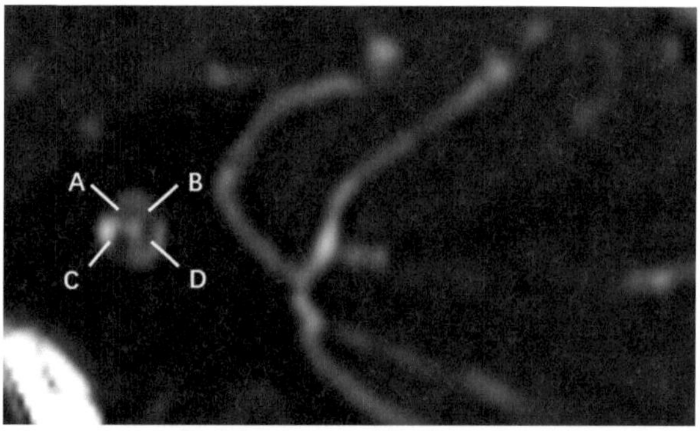

Fig. 4.1 High-resolution T2-weighted fast spin-echo MR images provide an excellent depiction of the intracanalicular segments of the facial nerve (FN) and the three divisions of the vestibulocochlear nerve in the oblique plane sagittal image obtained at the fundus of the internal auditory canal (IAC). (A) The facial nerve, (B) superior vestibular nerve, (C) cochlear nerve, and (D) inferior vestibular nerve

From these anatomical and magnetic resonance imaging techniques, we can tell which nerves are present and their relative dimensions. In 90% of normal cases, the cochlear nerve is larger than the superior and inferior vestibular nerves. The cochlear nerve is similar to or larger than the FN in 64% of subjects. In addition, 70% of patients have four nerves in a symmetrical relationship to the contralateral IAC (Kim et al. 1998). Furthermore, MRI can also evaluate the tissues of the inner ear.

So far, CND has been confirmed by MRI. If the cochlear nerve is significantly thinner than the FN in the IAC, it is diagnosed as cochlear dysplasia, and if the cochlear nerve is not found, it is defined as cochlear nerve aplasia (Fig. 4.2). As for the vestibulocochlear nerve (VCN) hypoplasia, Casselman et al. proposed the following classification method: type 1, VCN aplasia with IAC stenosis; type 2, a common VCN, with a hypoplastic or aplastic cochlear branch; and type 3, a common VCN with a hypoplastic or aplastic vestibular branch (Casselman et al. 1997). Another grading method for assessing cochlear nerve development is based on the number of nerves in the IAC. This method system included five grades. Grade 0 means no visible nerves in IAC, grade 1 means one nerve in IAC, and so on. Grade 4 means four nerves visible in the internal auditory canal, including hypoplastic nerves. Grade 5 represents the presence of four normal-sized nerves in IAC.

In a recent study by Han et al., the area, not the diameter, of the VCN was measured and correlated with the results of CI. They speculate that the VCN region may more accurately reflect the number of cochlear nerve fiber and then they compared VCN to FN ratios in IAC and CPA, which was used as a reference to diagnose cochlear nerve hypoplasia in IAC and CPA (Han et al. 2019). CND was recently shown to be one of the most common MRI findings in patients with auditory neuropathy spectrum disorder, which was shown to have normal function based on the presence of otoacoustic emissions or cochlear microphonics (Roche et al. 2010).

However, CND remains a diagnostic challenge. There are some limitations to MRI evaluation. First, it is difficult to differentiate cochlear nerve hypoplasia from cochlear nerve aplasia. We diagnosed cochlear nerve aplasia when it could not be identified on axial, coronal, or oblique sagittal MRI. If there are tiny nerves, care must be taken not to overinterpret the image as an absent nerve. However, an extremely small nerve below the limits of spatial resolution of MR imaging would

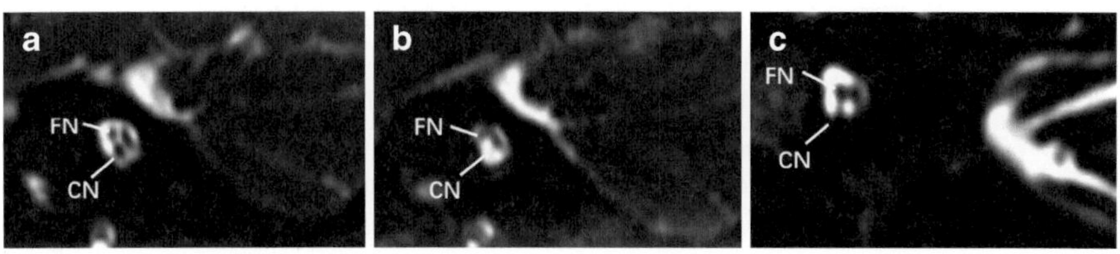

Fig. 4.2 High-resolution T2-weighted fast spin-echo MR images provide an excellent depiction of the facial nerve (FN) and vestibulocochlear nerve (VCN) in the internal auditory canal (IAC). (**a**) A child with unilateral deafness with normal FN and VCN in the right IAC. (**b**) The same case with Fig. **a**, the cochlear nerve within the left IAC is absent and is defined as cochlear nerve aplasia. (**c**) Another case with unilateral deafness, the cochlear nerve is significantly smaller than FN in IAC, which is considered cochlear nerve hypoplasia

appear absent. Song et al. showed the limitation of MRI in the diagnosis of nerve hypoplasia by revealing a thin but visible VCN during surgery in four cases, which had not been seen in preoperative MRI (Song et al. 2011). Therefore, in the broadest sense, cochlear nerve aplasia may contain an invisible nerve and one that is truly absent. Second, congenital and acquired degeneration of the cochlear nerve has been demonstrated by pathology (Ylikoski and Savolainen 1984; Felix and Hoffmann 1985; Spoendlin and Schrott 1990; Nadol Jr. and Xu 1992), while this cannot be differentiated on high-resolution MRI. There is no distinction between acquired degeneration resulting in a deficient nerve and the appearance of congenital neural deficiency. Third, the "mixed nerve" hypothesis has been proposed in which a thin or absent cochlear nerve intermingles with facial or vestibular nerve fibers and forms a "functionally combined" trunk that turns directly toward the cochlea (Buchman et al. 2011; Ozdoğmuş et al. 2004). This mixed nerve fibers in the IAC can transmit auditory information, allowing CND patients with CI to hear even have no CN presence in MRI (Ozdoğmuş et al. 2004; Tian et al. 2008). The "mixed nerve" has not been found on high-resolution T2-weighted MRI yet. Therefore, a thorough clinical evaluation including electrical stimulation is still important in selecting patients who may benefit from CI.

4.3 Correlation Between MRI Findings and CI Outcomes in Deafness with CND

CIs work by electrically stimulating spiral ganglion neurons. Electrical stimulation of CI is transmitted to the cochlear nucleus through the cochlear nerve (Zeng et al. 2008). The presence of the cochlear nerve plays an essential role in achieving ideal outcomes. The size of the cochlear nerve is considered correlated with the spiral ganglion cell population (Nadol Jr. and Xu 1992); determining the nerve caliber in cases of CND with high-resolution MR images may help predict the outcome of CI.

Generally, hearing outcomes after cochlear implantation are seldom satisfactory in children with CND. Some of them did not develop sufficient speech intelligibility (Walton et al. 2008; Kang et al. 2010; Kutz et al. 2011; Zhang et al. 2012), which means that the number of cochlear nerve fibers might be related to the outcome of CI in patients with CND, and the quantitative evaluation of the cochlear nerve might help predict speech performance after CI. The quantitative evaluation of the cochlear nerve size in IAC with MRI was difficult due to the limitation of image resolution and diverse aberrant course of the cochlear nerve in CND (Giesemann et al. 2012). The diameter of the cochlear nerve was reported to be correlated with the size of the VCN. The cochlear nerve is contained within the VCN, located in the CPA, just outside the midbrain. Therefore, the size of the VCN might indirectly represent the size of the cochlear nerve and spiral ganglion neurons (Nadol and Xu 1992). In a recent study, Han et al. proposed that the preoperative auditory brainstem response and area ratio of VCN to FN in CPA could predict CI outcomes in patients with CND (Han et al. 2019).

Regarding cochlear nerve aplasia, electrical stimulation with the CI electrode in the cochlear may theoretically not reach the brainstem and auditory cortex in patients (Maxwell et al. 1999), and it has always been considered an absolute contraindication to CI. However, recent studies have reported that children with cochlear nerve aplasia on MRI can also benefit from CI, and their auditory skills, sound awareness, and speech perception can improve after surgery (Casselman et al. 1997; Acker et al. 2001; Govaerts et al. 2003; Bradley et al. 2008; Oker et al. 2009; Kang et al. 2010; Warren et al. 2010; Buchman et al. 2011; Kutz et al. 2011; Young et al. 2012), and the response of auditory cortex to acoustic stimulation was identified although the cochlear nerve was absent in MR images (Thai-Van et al. 2000). Clearly, some nerve fibers were available to transmit auditory signals to the brainstem (Casselman et al. 1997; Ozdoğmuş et al. 2004).

Therefore, it could be hypothesized that the cochlear branch runs together with vestibular fibers into the vestibule or that there is pluripotence of cochlear nerve fibers (Schuknecht 1993). The ectopic location of cochlear nerve fibers close to the vestibule was proposed in a study by Jahan et al., who demonstrated, in a mouse model that exhibited a shortened and misshapen cochlea, that the spiral ganglion cells of the cochlear nerve can be found close to the vestibule (Jahan et al. 2010). These findings suggest that MRI probably visualizes cochlear nerve hypoplasia (as opposed to aplasia). Even the highly T2-weighted 3D-sequence falls far short of the capabilities of microscopy; if only a few nerve fibers are present, these might be unrecognized. This has been proven in a study that revealed a thin but visible VCN during surgery that was not observed on preoperative MRI (Song et al. 2011). Therefore, the MRI depiction of an absent cochlear nerve in IAC is the only relative contraindication to CI.

The potential association between preoperative MRI findings and CI outcomes in patients with CND has been investigated in several studies (Walton et al. 2008; Yamazaki et al. 2015). In theory, the size of the cochlear nerve rather than the VCN should provide an index of the number of spiral ganglion neurons. However, due to limited spatial resolution, thin cochlear nerves cannot be accurately assessed based on MRI images. A recent study revealed that the size of the VCN did not have a significant correlation with the outcome of CI in children with CND. In contrast, there was a significant correlation between the VCN/FN ratio and the CI outcomes. These results indicate that the VCN/FN ratio as a predictor could be more sensitive than the absolute diameter of the VCN in children with CND with the normal function of FN (Chao et al. 2016).

4.4 Conclusion

High-resolution T2-weighted fast spin-echo MR imaging can be used to depict CND in the IAC. Therefore, it is of great practical importance for operative consideration before CI. Consequently, an accurate preoperative MRI evaluation of CND plays a key role in selecting the optimal management strategy for these children. However, there are some limitations to MRI as a diagnostic approach for CND. The preoperative evaluation of CI requires a comprehensive consideration of imaging and clinical factors.

References

Acker T, Mathur NN, et al. Is there a functioning vestibulocochlear nerve? Cochlear implantation in a child with symmetrical auditory findings but asymmetric imaging. Int J Pediatr Otorhinolaryngol. 2001;57(2):171–6.

Bradley J, Beale T, et al. Variable long-term outcomes from cochlear implantation in children with hypoplastic auditory nerves. Cochlear Implants Int. 2008;9(1):34–60.

Buchman CA, Teagle HF, et al. Cochlear implantation in children with labyrinthine anomalies and cochlear nerve deficiency: implications for auditory brainstem implantation. Laryngoscope. 2011;121(9):1979–88.

Casselman JW, Offeciers FE, et al. Aplasia and hypoplasia of the vestibulocochlear nerve: diagnosis with MR imaging. Radiology. 1997;202(3):773.

Chao X, Luo J, et al. Usefulness of radiological findings for predicting cochlear implantation outcomes in children with cochlear nerve deficiency: a pilot study. Acta Otolaryngol. 2016;136(10):1051–7.

Clemmens CS, Guidi J, et al. Unilateral cochlear nerve deficiency in children. Otolaryngol Head Neck Surg. 2013;149(2):318–25.

Colletti L, Colletti G, Mandalà M, Colletti V. The Therapeutic dilemma of cochlear nerve deficiency. Otolaryngology–Head and Neck Surgery. 2014;151(2):308–14. https://doi.org/10.1177/0194599814531913.

Dagkiran M, Dagkiran N, et al. Radiological imaging findings of patients with congenital totally hearing loss. J Int Adv Otol. 2016;12:43–8.

Felix H, Hoffmann V. Light and electron microscopic investigation of cochlear nerve specimens from profoundly deaf patients. Acta Otolaryngol Suppl. 1985;423:67–72.

Giesemann AM, Kontorinis G, et al. The vestibulocochlear nerve: aplasia and hypoplasia in combination with inner ear malformations. Eur Radiol. 2012;22(3):519–24.

Glastonbury CM, Davidson HC, et al. Imaging findings of cochlear nerve deficiency. AJNR Am J Neuroradiol. 2002;23(4):635–43.

Govaerts PJ, Casselman J, et al. Cochlear implants in aplasia and hypoplasia of the cochleovestibular nerve. Otol Neurotol. 2003;24(6):887–91.

Han JJ, Suh MW, et al. A predictive model for cochlear implant outcome in children with cochlear nerve deficiency. Sci Rep. 2019;9(1):1154.

Held P, Fellner C, et al. MRI of inner ear anatomy using 3D MP-RAGE and 3D CISS sequences. Br J Radiol. 1997;70:465–72.

Herman B, Angeli S. Differences in cochlear nerve cross-sectional area between normal hearing and postlingually deafened patients on MRI. Otolaryngol Head Neck Surg. 2011;144:64–6.

Jahan I, Kersigo J, et al. Neurod1 regulates survival and formation of connections in mouse ear and brain. Cell Tissue Res. 2010;341:95–110.

Kang WS, Lee JH, et al. Cochlear implantations in young children with cochlear nerve deficiency diagnosed by MRI. Otolaryngol Head Neck Surg. 2010;143(1):101–8.

Kim HS, Kim DI, et al. Topographical relationship of the facial and vestibulocochlear nerves in the subarachnoid space and internal auditory canal. AJNR Am J Neuroradiol. 1998;19:1155–61.

Kutz JW Jr, Lee KH, et al. Cochlear implantation in children with cochlear nerve absence or deficiency. Otol Neurotol. 2011;32(6):956–61.

Lane JI, Ward H, et al. 3-T imaging of the cochlear nerve and labyrinth in cochlear-implant candidates: 3D fast recovery fast spin-echo versus 3D constructive interference in the steady state techniques. AJNR Am J Neuroradiol. 2004;25:618–22.

Lin PH, Hsu CJ, et al. Etiologic and audiologic characteristics of patients with pediatric-onset unilateral and asymmetric sensorineural hearing loss. JAMA Otolaryngol Head Neck Surgery. 2017;143:912–9.

Maxwell AP, Mason SM, et al. Cochlear nerve aplasia: its importance in cochlear implantation. Am J Otol. 1999;20:335–7.

Mcclay JE, Booth TN, et al. Evaluation of pediatric sensorineural hearing loss with magnetic resonance imaging. Arch Otolaryngol Head Neck Surg. 2008;134(9):945.

Nadol JB Jr, Xu WZ. Diameter of the cochlear nerve in deaf humans: implications for cochlear implantation. Ann Otol Rhinol Laryngol. 1992;101:988–93.

Nakano A, Arimoto Y, et al. Cochlear nerve deficiency and associated clinical features in patients with bilateral and unilateral hearing loss. Otol Neurotol. 2013;34(3):554–8.

Oker N, Loundon N, et al. Bilateral implantation in children with cochleovestibular nerve hypoplasia. Int J Pediatr Otorhinolaryngol. 2009;73(10):1470–3.

Ozdoğmuş O, Sezen O, et al. Connections between the facial, vestibular and cochlear nerve bundles within the internal auditory canal. J Anat. 2004;205(1):65–75.

Parry DA, Booth T, et al. Advantages of magnetic resonance imaging over computed tomography in preoperative evaluation of pediatric cochlear implant candidates. Otol Neurotol. 2005;26(5):976–82.

Roche JP, Huang BY, et al. Imaging characteristics of children with auditory neuropathy spectrum disorder. Otol Neurotol. 2010;31(5):780–8.

Rubinstein D, Sandberg EJ, et al. Anatomy of the facial and vestibulocochlear nerves in the internal auditory canal. AJNR Am J Neuroradiol. 1996;17:1099–105.

Peng KA, Kuan EC, Hagan S, Wilkinson EP, Miller ME. Cochlear nerve aplasia and hypoplasia: predictors of cochlear implant success. Otolaryngology–Head and Neck Surgery. 2017;157(3):392–400. https://doi.org/10.1177/0194599817718798.

Schuknecht HF. Pathology of the ear. 2nd ed. Pennsylvania: Lea & Febiger; 1993. 672 pp.

Song MH, Kim SC, et al. The cochleovestibular nerve identified during auditory brainstem implantation in patients with narrow internal auditory canals: can preoperative evaluation predict cochleovestibular nerve deficiency? Laryngoscope. 2011;121:1773–9.

Spoendlin H, Schrott A. Quantitative evaluation of the human cochlear nerve. Acta Otolaryngol Suppl. 1990;470:61–70.

Thai-Van H, Fraysse B, et al. Functional magnetic resonance imaging may avoid misdiagnosis of cochleovestibular nerve aplasia in congenital deafness. Otol Neurotol. 2000;21(5):663.

Tian GY, Xu DC, et al. The topographical relationships and anastomosis of the nerves in the human internal auditory canal. Surg Radiol Anat. 2008;30:243–7.

Usami SI, et al. Etiology of single-sided deafness and asymmetrical hearing loss. Acta Otolaryngol. 2017;137:S2–7.

Vesseur AR, Chantal F, et al. Hearing restoration in cochlear nerve deficiency: the choice between cochlear implant or auditory brainstem implant a meta-analysis. Otol Neurotol. 2018;39(4):428–37. https://doi.org/10.1097/MAO.0000000000001727.

Walton J, Gibson WP, et al. Predicting cochlear implant outcomes in children with auditory neuropathy. Otol Neurotol. 2008;29:302–9.

Warren FM 3rd, Wiggins RH 3rd, et al. Apparent cochlear nerve aplasia: to implant or not to implant? Otol Neurotol. 2010;31(7):1088–94.

Yamazaki H, Leigh J, et al. Usefulness of MRI and EABR testing for predicting CI Outcomes immediately after cochlear implantation in cases with cochlear nerve deficiency. Otol Neurotol. 2015;36:977–84.

Ylikoski J, Savolainen S. The cochlear nerve in various forms of deafness. Acta Otolaryngol. 1984;98:418–27.

Young NM, Kim FM, et al. Pediatric cochlear implantation of children with eighth nerve deficiency. Int J Pediatr Otorhinolaryngol. 2012;76(10):1442–8.

Zeng FG, Rebscher S, et al. Cochlear implants: system design, integration, and evaluation. IEEE Rev Biomed Eng. 2008;1:115–42.

Zhang Z, Li Y, et al. Cochlear implantation in children with cochlear nerve deficiency: a report of nine cases. Int J Pediatr Otorhinolaryngol. 2012;76:1188–95.

Preoperative Auditory and Electrophysiological Evaluation for Cochlear Nerve Deficiency

5

Shuo Wang, Jiong Hu, Jingyuan Chen, Simeng Lu, Xingmei Wei, and Yongxin Li

Cochlear nerve deficiency (CND) has a prevalence of approximately 6–28% in patients with auditory neuropathy spectrum disorder (ANSD) (Valero et al. 2012). It is also one of the main etiologies of congenital single-sided deafness (SSD) (Matsuura et al. 2022). In this section, we will provide a systematic review of audiological assessment in patients with CND. We will also discuss the evaluation of the outcome and prediction of cochlear implantation (CI) in patients with CND through electrically evoked auditory brainstem responses (EABR).

5.1 Audiological Characteristics of Patients with CND

CI evaluation typically involves audiological assessments, including pure tone audiometry, speech audiometry, immittance test battery, distortion product otoacoustic emissions (DPOAE), auditory brainstem response (ABR), auditory steady-state response (ASSR), and 40 Hz auditory evoked potential (40 Hz AEP).

S. Wang (✉)
Beijing Institute of Otolaryngology, Beijing Tongren Hospital, Capital Medical University, Beijing, China

Key Laboratory of Otolaryngology Head and Neck Surgery (Capital Medical University), Ministry of Education, Beijing, China

J. Hu
Department of Audiology, University of the Pacific, San Francisco, CA, USA
e-mail: jhu@PACIFIC.EDU

J. Chen · S. Lu · X. Wei · Y. Li
Key Laboratory of Otolaryngology Head and Neck Surgery (Capital Medical University), Ministry of Education, Beijing, China

Department of Otorhinolaryngology Head and Neck Surgery, Beijing Tongren Hospital, Capital Medical University, Beijing, China

Y. Li (ed.), *Cochlear Implantation for Cochlear Nerve Deficiency*,
https://doi.org/10.1007/978-981-19-5892-2_5

5.1.1 Pure Tone Audiometry

Patients with CND typically have severe to profound sensorineural hearing loss (SNHL). In 2020, Fan et al. (2020) reported an average threshold of 110.00 ± 9.01 dB HL at 1000 Hz in patients with absent cochlear nerve (20 ears). They also reported an average threshold of 100.00 ± 13.36 dB HL at 1000 Hz in patients with cochlear nerve hypoplasia (10 ears). Matsuura et al. (2022) reported an average hearing threshold of 92.4 ± 17.65 dB HL in 61 patients with CND, of which 88% were those with severe to profound hearing loss. Cinar et al. reported that in 66 patients with cochlear nerve hypoplasia (112 ears), 59.3% had severe to profound hearing loss, while 23.5% had no response to sound (Cinar et al. 2017).

Limited research has been conducted on different audiogram configurations of patients with CND. Matsuura et al. (2022) categorized audiograms from patients with CND into three configurations: flat (78.7%), U-shaped (9.8%), and sloping (9.8%). They also noted that there seemed to be no relationship between the type of CND and the audiogram configurations of the patients. In 2015, Zhang et al. (2015) (Buchman et al. 2006) reported that among four patients with CND, two had flat audiograms, one had a rising audiogram, and the last had a sloping configuration.

5.1.2 Pediatric Audiometry

Similarly to the thresholds obtained from adult pure tone audiometry, pediatric patients with CND often provide severe to profound behavioral thresholds (Fig. 5.1). In 2006, Buchman et al. (2006) examined the audiological characteristics of nine

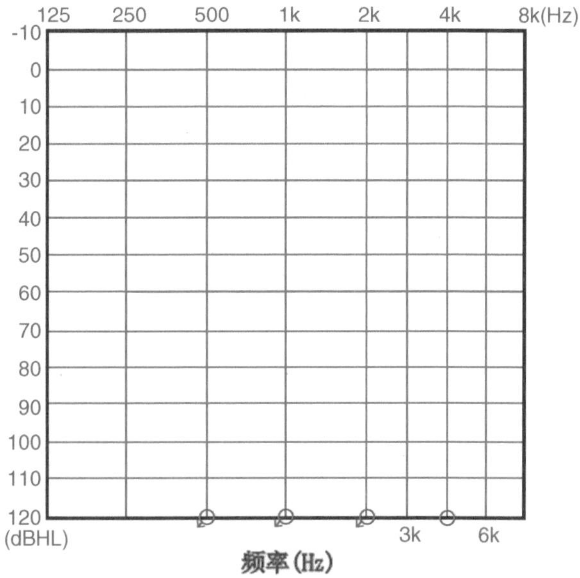

Fig. 5.1 Pediatric audiometry on the right side of a pediatric patient with CND

pediatric patients with CND. They obtained behavioral thresholds from five of them (eight ears), all of whom had severe to profound hearing losses. Clemmens et al. (2013) investigated 128 pediatric patients with SNHL; they found 33 patients with CND by audiological assessment and imaging, of whom 24 (72.7%) had severe to profound hearing losses. Our center summarized the results of pediatric audiometry in 73 patients with CND with normal cochlea and 67 patients with CND with severe inner ear malformation (IEM) before CI. If no measurable response was assumed to be 5 dB HL greater than the maximum output of the audiometer (120 dB HL), which was 125 dB HL. Among them, the mean residual hearing in patients with CND with normal cochlea was 108.05 ± 14.63 dB HL, ranging from 81.25 to 125.00 dB HL. The mean residual hearing in patients with CND with severe IEM was 120.78 ± 9.81 dB HL, ranging from 80.00 to 125.00 dB HL.

5.1.3 Speech Audiometry

Speech perception and recognition ability in patients with CND are lower than in those with intact cochlear nerves. Zhang et al. (Cinar et al. 2017) examined four patients with CND (seven ears) in whom their speech recognition rates were lower than 40%, two of whom had a score of 0%. In 2008, Walton et al. (2008) examined 54 patients with ANSD and found that those with CND had significantly lower word recognition scores than those without CND. Yousef et al. (2021) examined post-implantation speech awareness thresholds (SAT) obtained from pediatric patients and reported that children in the control group had significantly higher SATs than those with cochlear nerve hypoplasia or deficiency. Poor speech cognition ability in patients with CND could be due to the dyssynchrony of neural firing resulting from developmental abnormalities of the auditory nerve.

5.1.4 Immittance Test Battery

Tympanograms obtained from patients with CND are typically type A or type As, with absent acoustic reflexes. Zhang et al. (Cinar et al. 2017) reported seven type A tympanograms and one type As tympanogram in four patients with CND (seven ears), none of whom had acoustic reflexes. In the 30 patients reported by Fan et al. (2020), types A, As, Ad, B, and C tympanograms were reported at 38.9%, 40.7%, 3.7%, 7.4%, and 7.4%, respectively, in which all patients with types B and C tympanograms had middle ear pathologies. In our center, types A, As, Ad, B, and C tympanograms of patients with CND who underwent CI were 72.9%, 20.0%, 0%, 3.6%, and 4.9%, respectively. The difference may be because our patients are all CI candidates and severe middle ear pathologies were excluded.

5.1.5 Otoacoustic Emissions

DPOAE can be present in patients with CND, which is a retrocochlear pathology. Zhang et al. (Cinar et al. 2017) reported that all four patients with CND had DPOAE at almost all frequencies. In the 30 patients reported by Fan et al. (2020), six patients had DPOAE at all or some frequency in one or both ears. Matsuura et al. (2022) examined 61 patients with unilateral CND and reported that 9.8% (6 patients) had DPOAE at some frequencies, and their DPOAE persisted during follow-up. In our center, 3.6% of patients with CND who underwent CI had DPOAE. These results indicate that some cases of CND are clinically diagnosed with ANSD. Some studies also suggested that unilateral ANSD with profound hearing loss should be highly indicative of CND diagnosis (Buchman et al. 2006; Liu et al. 2012).

5.1.6 ABR and Cochlear Microphonic

Patients with CND are typically expected to have severely abnormal or absent ABR. However, cochlear microphonic (CM) can be found in some patients with CND, as CND can be considered a retrocochlear pathology. Buchman et al. (2006) examined nine pediatric patients with CND (13 ears), of whom none had a click or tone-burst-evoked ABR, while nine ears had CM. Liu et al. (2012) investigated eight patients with single-sided CND through 100 us clicks; they found that only one patient had ABR, with a threshold at 97 dB nHL, while all patients had CM present. In 2020, Lu et al. (2020) reported that in seven patients with CND (two unilateral and five bilateral), only one patient with bilateral CND had ABR at 90 dB nHL on the patient's left side. In our center, only 2.85% of patients with CND had ABR and 5.0% had CM before CI.

5.1.7 Other Auditory Evoked Potentials

Currently, studies on ASSR (Fig. 5.2) and 40 Hz AEP in patients with CND are limited. ASSR is known for its frequency specificity and is used to estimate behavioral thresholds in infants and young children. Fan et al. (2020) obtained averaged thresholds between 0.5 and 4 kHz in patients with CND that are consistent with their pure tone audiometry results. They also reported that patients with absent cochlear nerves had worse ASSR thresholds than those with cochlear nerve hypoplasia at all frequencies. This is consistent with the data in our center. Most of patients with CND had absent ASSR responses as shown in Fig. 5.2.

The 40 Hz AEP has been used as an objective evaluation tool to assess low-frequency hearing in adults and older children. Lu et al. (2020) reported that in seven patients with CND evaluated with 40 Hz AEP, all thresholds were obtained at 90–110 dB nHL, with no responses from three ears, which was consistent with their behavioral thresholds. Approximately 20% of patients with CND undergoing CI at our center had responses in 40 Hz AEP.

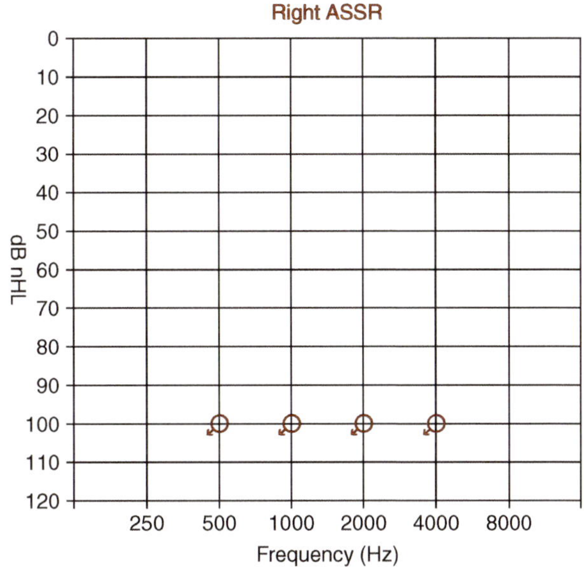

Fig. 5.2 The right side's ASSR of a pediatric patient with CND

5.2 Applications of EABR

The assessment of outcomes and the prediction of CI are difficult in patients with CND through pre-surgical EABRs. Previous studies used EABR and electrically evoked auditory nerve compound action potentials (ECAP) before, during, and after CI, to assess the site of implantation and predict its outcome.

5.2.1 EABR

EABR evaluates the response of the auditory system to an electrical signal by stimulating the cochlear. It approximates the working scenario of CI and can be used as a more accurate estimation tool for the prediction of implantation outcomes (Kileny and Zwolan 2004; Nicolas et al. 2016). Clinically, it is typical to obtain EABR by stimulating with an external electrode and recording responses from the cochlear nerve before and during the CI surgery or by stimulating with an internal electrode of the CI after surgery. Pre- and peri-surgical EABR are more clinically valuable as they can provide information on the status, as well as the integrity and function of the CI recipient's auditory system (Wang et al. 2016). Kileny et al. (1987) described the utility of EABR in the pre-surgical CI evaluation. They suggested that EBAR could help select the side of implantation in children with anatomical abnormalities and help evaluate the cochlear nerve status. A review study by Warren et al. (2015) in 2010 suggested that EBAR, together with imaging modalities, can provide valuable information in assessing the residual functionality of the cochlear nerve. Wang et al. (2016) suggested that EABR can investigate the physiological responses of the auditory system under electrical stimulation by electronically stimulating the cochlear. It estimates the functioning status of the working cochlear and thus can be used to predict the prognosis of implantation patients more accurately. Birman et al. (2016) suggested that trans-tympanic EBAR can help select the implantation side and that CI electrode-evoked EBAR can be used to assess the integrity of the cochlear nerve. However, because trans-tympanic EBAR is invasive and has a low elicitation rate, it is now rarely used. Yamazaki et al. (2015) investigated pediatric patients with CND and reported that the diameters of the facial nerve and vestibulocochlear nerve were examined by pre-surgical MRI and whether peri-surgical EABR wave V was present was highly correlated with patients' prognosis and speech-language development. In a study by Huang et al. (2019), pre-surgical imaging and EABR measurements were analyzed in six pediatric patients with CND with single-sided implantation, along with examination of the patients' post-surgical audiological assessment and speech-language evaluation. They found that comprehensive pre-surgical electrophysiological evaluation in pediatric patients with CND can more accurately assess the integrity of the auditory pathway and evaluate functions of the cochlear nerve and provide important information in deciding whether to proceed with surgery. Minami et al. (2021) classified pediatric patients with CND and measured their EABR. The Minami classification system is based on modiolus deficiency and the internal auditory canal cochlear nerve and grades I to IV. Grade I is defined as modiolus present and normal cochlear nerve; Grade II is defined as modiolus deficiency and normal cochlear nerve; Grade III is defined as modiolus present and CND; Grade IV is defined as modiolus deficiency and CND. Their results suggested that the percentages of present EABR in the different classifications are: 93%, 36%, 23%, and 50% for Classes I, II, III, and IV, respectively. Class I CND had a significantly higher percentage of present EABR than the other groups, confirming the utility of EABR in assessing pediatric patients with CND. In our center, if a patient with CND cannot elicit any residual hearing and EABR cannot also be elicited, auditory training with a hearing aid will be performed to determine the function of the cochlear nerve. Training details have been introduced in our previous book (Li 2022).

In our center, we also performed EABR before and during CI surgery for some patients with CND and will share the experience and results below. We used PromStim (Promontory Stimulation) to elicit EABR, which is a tool to stimulate the cochlea before or during the CI surgery described by Kuo and Gibson in 2002 (Kuo and Gibson 2010). EABR could be stimulated using a PromStim electrode before or during CI surgery or a CI electrode after CI surgery. Although the results of the two above methods are not completely identical, both may help predict CI outcomes. The stimulation electrode (PromStim electrode) is a temporary needle placed in different positions when testing EABR before or during CI surgery based on whether it is associated with a cochlear deformity (Polterauer et al. 2017, 2018). For patients with normal cochlear structures, we place the stimulation electrode in the promontory, and when the patient has a common cavity deformity, we usually open the cavity and place the stimulation electrodes at the bottom of the common cavity; this method was mentioned in our previous book (Li 2022).

A total of 13 patients were tested, nine of whom had common cavity deformity (CCD), and the remaining had normal cochlear structures with or without bony cochlear nerve canal (BCNC) stenosis. Of the nine patients, five elicited EABR waves before CI and four elicited EABR waves after CI (Table 5.1). According to Minami's grading, 50% (2/4) of Grade III and 66.7% (6/9) of Grade IV patients at our center showed EABR waves, compared to 23% and 50%, respectively, in their study (Minami et al. 2021). However, EABR waves were elicited by the PromStim electrode before CI surgery or by the CI electrode after CI surgery in our center, while EABR waves were elicited by the CI electrode in the study by Minami.

Our results showed that EABR was elicited during the CI surgery test in some patients, but not after implantation. We believe that this phenomenon is mainly related to the location of electrode stimulation, especially in patients with common cavity malformations, and whether the electrodes attached to the lateral wall of the cavity after surgery may affect these results. We believe that intracochlear EABRs are more meaningful for patients with normal cochlear structures, while EABRs before CI surgery may be influenced by interference and stimulus location. The prediction of CI outcomes using EABR results requires long-term observation with a large sample size. There are three cases of pediatric patients with CI.

Case 1: A 2-year-old boy with normal cochlear structures, stenotic IAC, and BCNC (Fig. 5.3a, b), who underwent CI surgery (Cochlear, Australia) in his left ear in 2020. EABR waves were elicited by CI electrodes (Fig. 5.3c).

Case 2: A 5-year-old boy with normal cochlear structures (Fig. 5.4a) and narrow IAC (Fig. 5.4b) underwent CI surgery (MED-EL) in his right ear in 2022 (Fig. 5.4c). EABR waves are elicited in the right ear by CI electrodes (Fig. 5.4d).

Table 5.1 Clinical data from 13 patients

No.	Age	Sex	Side	cochlea	IAC	BCNC	EABR before CI	EABR after CI
1 ANSD	7M	Female	Left	Normal		Stenosis	(−)	(−)
2	10M	Male	Left	Normal		Stenosis	(−)	(−)
3 (Case1)	2Y	Male	Left	Normal	Narrow	Stenosis	/	(+)
4 (Case2)	5Y	Male	Right	Normal	Narrow	Normal	/	(+)
5	18Y	Male	Left	CCD		/	(−)	(−)
6	1Y	Female	Right	CCD		/	(−)	(+)
7 (Case3)	1Y	Female	Right	CCD		/	(+)	(+)
8	9M	Male	Left	CCD		/	(+)	(−)
9	1Y	Female	Right	CCD		/	(+)	(−)
10	3Y	Male	Right	CCD		/	(−)	(−)
11	1Y	Male	Right	CCD		/	Yes	No
12	1Y	Male	Left	CCD		/	No	No
13	1Y	Female	Left	CCD		/	Yes	No

BCNC Bony cochlear nerve canal, *IAC* internal auditory canal, *CCD* common cavity deformity

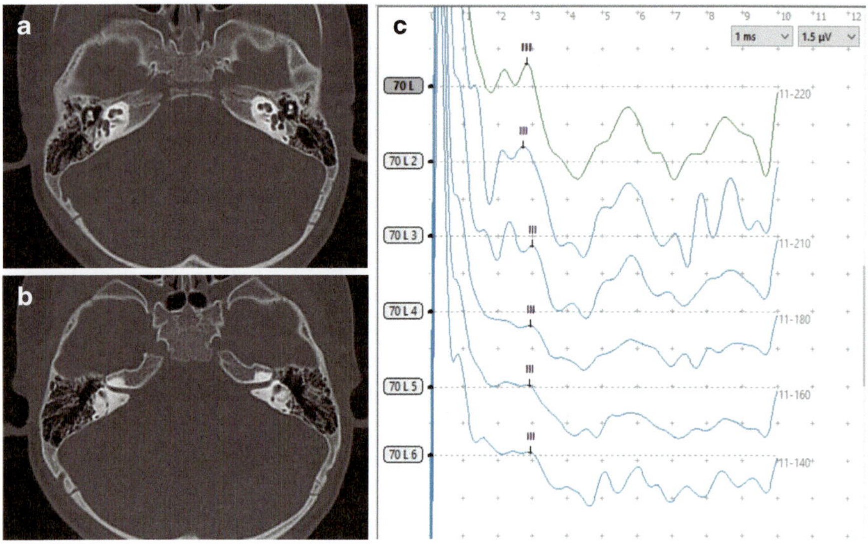

Fig. 5.3 The CT and EABR of case 1. (**a**) Bilateral BCNCs exhibit stenotic in axial HRCT. (**b**) Bilateral IACs exhibit stenotic on axial HRCT. (**c**) EABRs at different levels (positive III is elicited at electrode No. 11)

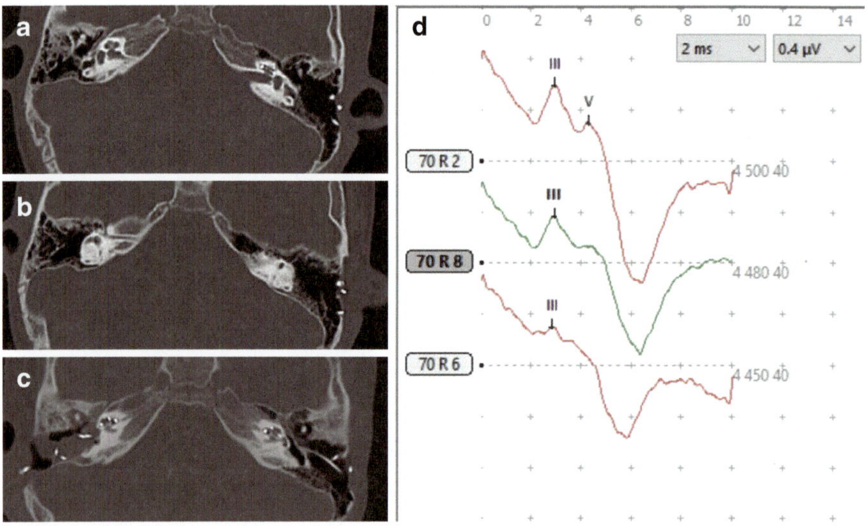

Fig. 5.4 CT and EABR of case 2. (**a**) Normal cochlea structure was shown on axial HRCT. (**b**) The right IAC exhibits stenotic in axial HRCT. (**c**) The post-operative image was shown on axial HRCT. (**d**) EABRs at different levels (positive III and V are elicited at electrode No. 4)

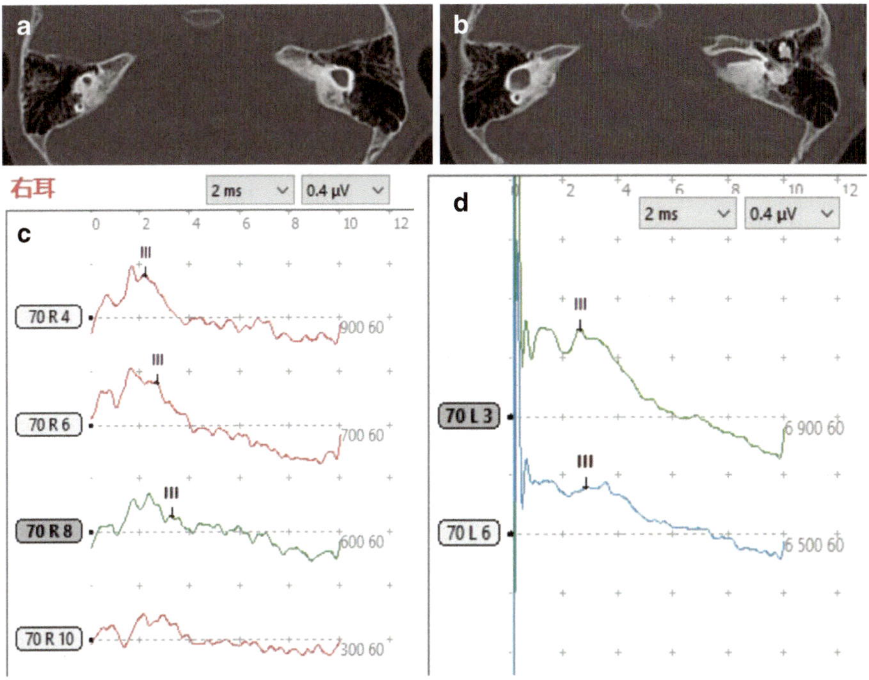

Fig. 5.5 CT and EABR of case 3. (**a**, **b**) CCD was shown on axial HRCT. (**c**) EABRs before CI surgery (positive III is elicited). (**d**) EABRs after CI surgery (positive III is elicited in electrode No. 6)

Case 3: A 1-year-old girl with CCD (Fig. 5.5a, b) underwent CI surgery (MED-EL) with a transmastoid slotted labyrinthotomy approach (TSLA) in her right ear in 2022. EABR waves are elicited in the right ear by the PromStim electrode and the CI electrode (Fig. 5.5c, d).

5.2.2 ECAP

ECAP generates and records the action potential from electrical stimulation of the spiral ganglion. It uses the “reversal” ability of CI to detect and assess the near-field responses of the cochlear nerve. Current research focuses more on obtaining ECAP thresholds through CI electrodes after implantation. Studies on ECAP in pediatric patients with CND are limited to this point.

He et al. suggested that ECAP can directly assess neural responses from the cochlear nerve and better reflect the functional status of the nerve, and its responses correlate with speech and perception abilities (He et al. 2012). ECAP can be detected in some children with confirmed CND, suggesting that residual neural fibers might remain in these children. He et al. (Shuman et al. 2019) further used ECAP to assess the functional status of cochlear nerves in children with CND; they suggested that discrepancies in previous ECAP literature should not reduce its utility in this particular group of patients. The functional status of the cochlear nerve in children with CND changes when the lengths of their cochlear differ. The ECAP thresholds for children with CND were significantly higher than those with a typically developed cochlear nerve. As the stimulating electrode shifts from the basal end to the apical end, the damage to the cochlear nerve worsens and the percentage of test electrodes that can be used to assess ECAP decreases. They also suggested that there appeared to be a relationship between the prolonged neural refractory period in the cochlear nerve and the slow stimulation rate used in the post-implantation adjustment. Luo et al. (2018) examined the amount of stimulation needed in the cochlear nerve of patients with CND and its functional status in a different section of the cochlear by evaluating ECAP and its threshold in both patients with CND and the control group; consistent with the report by He et al. (Shuman et al. 2019), Luo et al. found that more electrical stimulation is needed to evoke responses from the cochlear nerve in patients with CND. Furthermore, it was reported that in patients with cochlear nerve hypoplasia, lower cochlear nerve functionality was found in the low-frequency region, which also required a greater amount of electrical stimulation than in the higher-frequency regions of the cochlear.

For audiologists, CI mapping can be challenging due to the difficulty in obtaining reliable behavioral responses in patients with CND. Measuring ECAPs allows us to objectively verify cochlear nerve function stimulated by CI. ECAP could usually be detected in patients with normal cochlea structure and cochlear nerve function, but in children with CND, it is difficult to measure ECAP under regular parameters due to the small number of cochlear nerve fibers. He et al. (2020) found that ECAP could be easily detected by adjusting the stimulation and recording parameters. Due to the large variability of cochlear nerve function in patients with CND, the adjustment of the parameters varies between individuals. It is not recommended to measure ECAP intraoperatively with different parameters due to the long time required. We will share a case whose ECAP was elicited by adjusting the parameters in Chap. 7.

In summary, electrophysiological evaluations are important assessment tools in the examination of cochlear nerve function. They may supplement imaging modalities in pre-implantation evaluation and peri-surgical monitoring of patients with CND. They may also provide information on the prediction of aural rehabilitation outcomes in patients with CND after CI implantation.

References

Birman CS, Powell HRF, et al. Cochlear implant outcomes in cochlea nerve aplasia and hypoplasia. Otol Neurotol. 2016;37(5):438.

Buchman CA, Roush PA, et al. Auditory neuropathy characteristics in children with cochlear nerve deficiency. Ear Hear. 2006;27(4):399–408.

Cinar BC, Batuk MO, et al. Audiologic and radiologic findings in cochlear hypoplasia. Auris Nasus Larynx. 2017;44(6):655–63.

Clemmens CS, Guidi J, et al. Unilateral cochlear nerve deficiency in children. Otolaryngol Head Neck Surg. 2013;149(2):318–25.

Fan X, Lin Y, Ren C, Tang Y, Zha D. Auditory characteristics in patients with cochlear nerve deficiency[J]. Journal of Audiology and Speech Pathology. 2020;28(1):15–8.

He S, Grose J, et al. Cochlear implant-evoked cortical activation in children with cochlear nerve deficiency. Otol Neurotol. 2012;33(7):1188–96.

He S, Chao X, et al. Recommendations for measuring the electrically evoked compound action potential in children with cochlear nerve deficiency. Ear Hear. 2020;41(3):465–75.

Huang Y, Cheng L, et al. Preoperative imaging and electrophysiological evaluation of cochlear implantation in children with cochlear nerve dysplasia. J Clin Otorhinolaryngol Head Neck Surg. 2019;33(8):729–35.

Kileny PR, Zwolan TA. Pre-perioperative, transtympanic electrically evoked auditory brainstem response in children. Int J Audiol. 2004;43(Suppl 1):S16–21.

Kileny PR, et al. Electrically evoked middle-latency auditory potentials in cochlear implant candidates. Arch Otolaryngol Head Neck Surg. 1987;113(10):1072–7.

Kuo SC, Gibson WP. The role of the promontory stimulation test in cochlear implantation. Cochlear Implants Int. 2010;3(1):19–28.

Li Y. Cochlear implantation for common cavity deformity. Cham: Springer; 2022.

Liu C, Bu X, et al. Unilateral auditory neuropathy caused by cochlear nerve deficiency. Int J Otolaryngol. 2012;2012:1–5. https://doi.org/10.1155/2012/914986.

Lu Z, Pan T, et al. Imaging and audiological characteristics of patients with cochlear nerve dysplasia. Acta Anat Sin. 2020;5(51):693–8.

Luo J, Zhao X, et al. Auditory nerve responses after cochlear implantation in patients with cochlear nerve deficiency. Chin J Otol. 2018;16(6):816–21.

Matsuura K, Yoshimura H, et al. Audiological features in 63 patients with cochlear nerve deficiency. Otol Neurotol. 2022;43(1):23–8.

Minami SB, Yamamoto N, et al. Cochlear implantation in cases of inner ear malformation: a novel and simple grading, intracochlear EABR, and outcomes of hearing. Otol Neurotol. 2021;42:e117–23.

Nicolas G, Michel H, et al. A cochlear implant performance prognostic test based on electrical field interactions evaluated by eABR (Electrical Auditory Brainstem Responses). PLoS One. 2016;11(5):e0155008.

Polterauer D, Mandruzzato G, et al. Feasibility of promontory stimulation eABR recording in cochlear implant candidates with MED-EL clinical system. HNO-Kongress. 2017.

Polterauer D, Neuling M, et al. PromBERA: a preoperative eABR: an update. Curr Dir Biomed Eng. 2018;4(1):563–5.

Shuman L, et al. The effect of interphase gap on neural response of the electrically stimulated cochlear nerve in children with cochlear nerve deficiency and children with normal-sized cochlear nerves. Ear Hear. 2019;41(4):918–34.

Valero J, Blaser S, et al. Electrophysiologic and behavioral outcomes of cochlear implantation in children with auditory nerve hypoplasia. Ear Hear. 2012;33(1):3.

Walton J, Gibson W, et al. Predicting cochlear implant outcomes in children with auditory neuropathy. Otol Neurotol. 2008;29(3):302–9.

Wang B, Cao KL, et al. [Detection of the electric brain stem auditory response before cochlear implantation and its significance]. Zhonghua Er Bi Yan Hou Tou Jing Wai Ke Za Zhi = Chin J Otorhinolaryngol Head Neck Surg. 2016;51(11):826.

Warren FM, Wiggins RH, et al. Apparent cochlear nerve aplasia: to implant or not to implant? Otol Neurotol. 2015;31(7):1088–94.

Yamazaki H, Leigh J, et al. Usefulness of MRI and EABR testing for predicting CI outcomes immediately after cochlear implantation in cases with cochlear nerve deficiency. Otol Neurotol. 2015;36:977–84.

Yousef M, Mesallam TA, et al. Audiologic outcome of cochlear implantation in children with cochlear nerve deficiency. Otol Neurotol. 2021;42:38–46.

Zhang J, Zhang Q, Qi Y, Lan L, Yu L, Li N, Wang D, Wang Q. The radiological characteristics of cochlear nerve in patients with auditory neuropathy spectrum disorder[J]. Chin J Otol. 2015;2:242–5.

Cochlear Implantation Strategies and Techniques for Cochlear Nerve Deficiency Patients

6

Xingmei Wei, Simeng Lu, Shujin Xue, Biao Chen, Jingyuan Chen, Danmo Cui, Ying Shi, and Yongxin Li

6.1 Introduction

Nowadays, cochlear nerve deficiency (CND) is an indication for cochlear implantation (CI). However, the method to select the implantation side and electrode needs to be explored since embryonic development, residual hearing, and support from the patients' family are all factors that affect the selection process. In our center, nearly 300 CND patients underwent CI surgery and they were followed up regularly, so we have relatively abundant experience with this kind of cases. Next, we will discuss the CI strategies for CND patients under different circumstances.

6.2 CND without Inner Ear Malformation

About 70% of the CND patients do not have inner ear malformation (IEM) (Morlet et al. 2017). In our database, about 55% of CND patients who underwent CI had normal cochlea.

For severe bilateral sensorineural hearing loss patients with normal cochlea, if one side has CND, we undoubtedly select the side without CND as the implant side.

For bilateral CND patients with bilateral normal cochlea, we usually select the implant side according to their residual hearing and the nerve condition in the internal auditory canal (IAC). CND can be classified into 0 to III grades according to the number of nerve bundles in the IAC (Birman et al. 2016). The side with better residual hearing and more nerve bundles will be selected as the implant

X. Wei · S. Lu · S. Xue · B. Chen · J. Chen · D. Cui · Y. Shi · Y. Li (✉)
Department of Otorhinolaryngology Head and Neck Surgery, Beijing Tongren Hospital, Capital Medical University, Beijing, China

Key Laboratory of Otolaryngology Head and Neck Surgery (Capital Medical University), Ministry of Education, Beijing, China

Y. Li (ed.), *Cochlear Implantation for Cochlear Nerve Deficiency*,
https://doi.org/10.1007/978-981-19-5892-2_6

side. In clinical practice, the residual hearing is often consistent with the nerve bundles, that is, the more the nerve bundles in IAC, the better the residual hearing. If they are not consistent, we should find out where does the problem lie, and assess whether the hearing test results are genuine. If the number of nerve bundles on bilateral sides is the same, the residual hearing should be the main selection basis. For example, there was one patient with bilateral CND and there was only one nerve bundle each on both sides in the IAC (Fig. 6.1), and behavior audiometry showed that the left side had residual hearing but the right side had no detectable hearing, so we selected the left side for CI surgery. In addition, the cochlear aperture is an important structure to determine the implant side, because the one with CND is often accompanied with cochlear aperture stenosis, and the degree of cochlear aperture stenosis can reflect the diameter of the cochlear nerve (Orzan et al. 2021). For example, there was a patient with bilateral cochlear aperture stenosis and the CT showed that her right cochlear aperture was a little wider than the left one (Fig. 6.2a). The MRI also showed that her right side had three nerve bundles and the left side had two (Fig. 6.2b, c), and her residual hearing thresholds were also better on the right side than on the left side (average 90 dB HL & 100 dB HL), so we performed CI for her right side. However, if one side has auditory neuropathy (AN), we should avoid to select the AN side, because the CI results of AN patients are usually poor (Shearer and Hansen 2019). It is worth noting that for bilateral CND, bilateral CI at the same time should be avoided, because we have no idea whether the patients will get meaningful auditory ability after CI. After the implantation on one side is completed and the outcome is confirmed, then implanting the other side is recommended. In recent years, the vestibular function is also as a reference for side selection before CI (Coudert et al. 2017). If a patient's bilateral hearing and radiology parameters have no significant difference, the side with worse vestibular function can be selected as the implant side. The detailed information about vestibula function for CND will be introduced in Chap. 9.

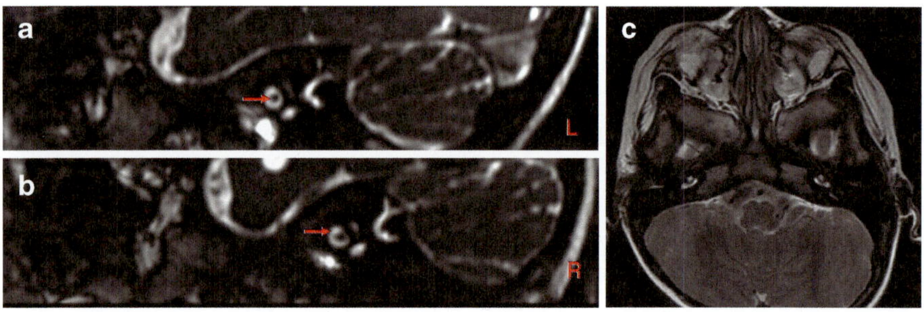

Fig. 6.1 (**a**, **b**). The left (**a**) and right (**b**) sides of oblique sagittal magnetic resonance imaging (MRI) of the inner ear show that there was one nerve bundle in the IAC. The red arrow points to the nerve bundle. (**c**) The T2 of MRI shows that the cochlea was normal

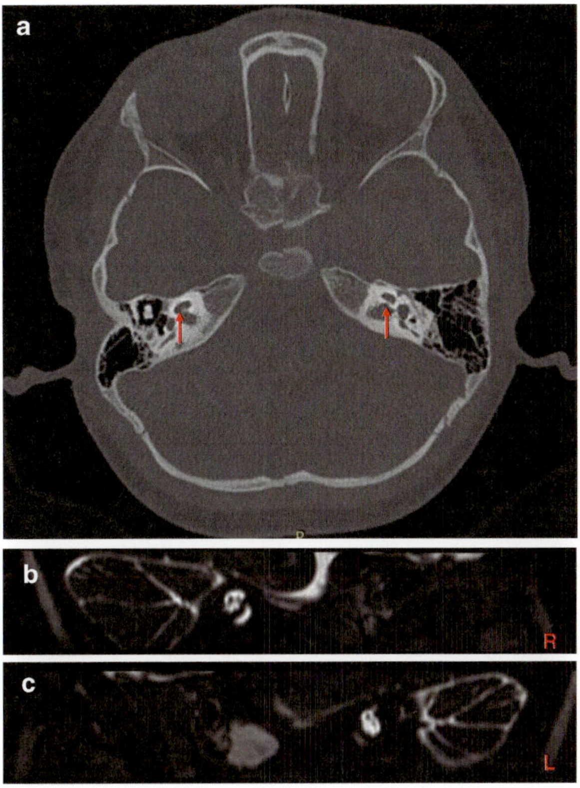

Fig. 6.2 (**a**) The temporal bone computed tomography (CT) shows bilaterally stenosed cochlear apertures, and the right one was a little wider than the left one. The red arrow points to the cochlear aperture. (**b**). The three nerve bundles in the right IAC. (**c**) The two nerve bundles in the left IAC

6.3 CND with Inner Ear Malformation

CND is related to anomalies of the cochlea (27%) and vestibule (49%) (Morlet et al. 2017). Therefore, there are many CND patients with IEM. For CI surgery, we mainly focus on cochlear structure.

According to the classification by Sennaroglu et al. (Sennaroğlu and Bajin 2017) in 2017, the cochlear malformation mainly included rudimentary otocyst (RO), cochlear aplasia (CA), common cavity deformity (CCD), cochlear hypoplasia (CH), incomplete partition type I (IP-I), incomplete partition type II (IP-II), and incomplete partition type III (IP-III). All these malformations can undergo CI surgery under some circumstances. RO, CA, CCD, CH, IP-I, and IP-II can accompany with CND, and we will introduce them below one by one.

6.3.1 Rudimentary Otocyst

RO is a more severe malformation than CCD and CA but better than Michel deformity. Since patients with RO have no internal auditory canal (IAC) formed (Sennaroğlu and Bajin 2017), they usually need an auditory brainstem implant

(ABI) to obtain sound (Ertugrul et al. 2021). However, in our case series, there was a one-year-old girl with RO in her right side and Michel malformation in her left side and she had no IAC bilaterally (Fig. 6.3a, b). After auditory training, she could respond to sound, and her parents desired to try CI for her. Therefore, we performed CI surgery for her with a transmastoid slotted labyrinthotomy approach (TSLA) (Wei et al. 2018) using customized electrodes (Med-EL, Sonata). The postoperative CT showed that the electrodes were almost all in the otocyst except for one electrode (Fig. 6.3c, d). One and a half years after surgery, her CAP, SIR, MAIS, and MUSS scores were 5, 2, 30, and 22, respectively, she could detect all the Ling-6 sounds, and the close-set speech showed that the mean disyllabic test score was 66.7%. Our experience demonstrated that even in cases of RO without IAC, there may be some cochlear nerve bundles existing which can be detected by present radiology.

6.3.2 Cochlear Aplasia

CA is a malformation that is better than RO but more severe than CCD, which is the lack of a cochlea with an existing IAC, vestibule, and superior semicircular canal (Sennaroğlu and Bajin 2017). CA usually has a dilated vestibule, which makes it easy to be confused with CCD. We usually consider that patients with CA are not fit for CI, because there is no cochlear nerve in the vestibule. However, based on our experience at our center, since the malformation is classified based on radiological findings, there are some nerve fibers that may not appear in the radiological images but the patients can perceive sound from the invisible nerve fibers. Below, we have shared one such case.

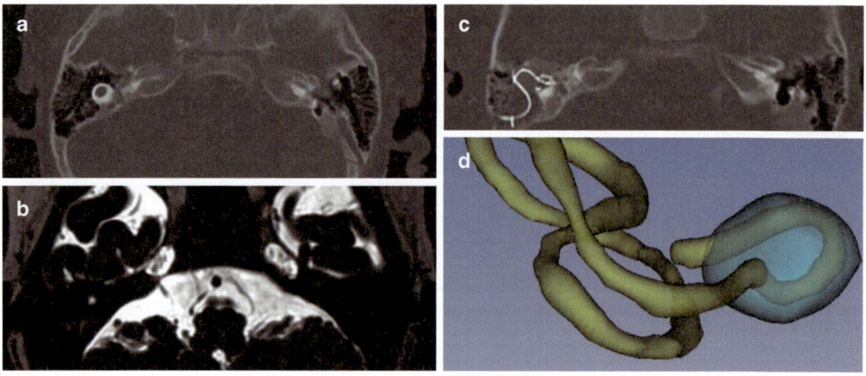

Fig. 6.3 (**a**) The CT shows that the patient's right side had RO, and her left side had Michel malformation. (**b**) The MRI shows that there was no IAC and cochlear neve. (**c**) Postoperative electrode shown in CT. (**d**) The three-dimensional (3D) image of the postoperative electrode

One two-year-old girl had CA, which could have easily been mistaken for RO because there was no routine IAC observed in CT, but a narrow slot could be found connecting the otocyst and brain (Fig. 6.4a). The inner ear MRI revealed that there were no cochlear nerve bundles in the IAC (Fig. 6.4b, c), but she could elicit objective hearing in her right ear. We performed CI surgery by TSLA (Wei et al. 2018) using customized electrodes (Med-EL, Concerto) for the patient (Fig. 6.4d). The postoperative CT showed that the electrodes were closely attached to the wall of the otocyst (Fig. 6.4e, f). One and a half year after surgery, she could understand common phrases without lip reading (CAP = 4), her speech comprised single words (SIR = 2), she had good detection and responded to environmental sounds and signals (IT-MAIS = 32), and she could use speech frequently (MUSS = 6). She was able to

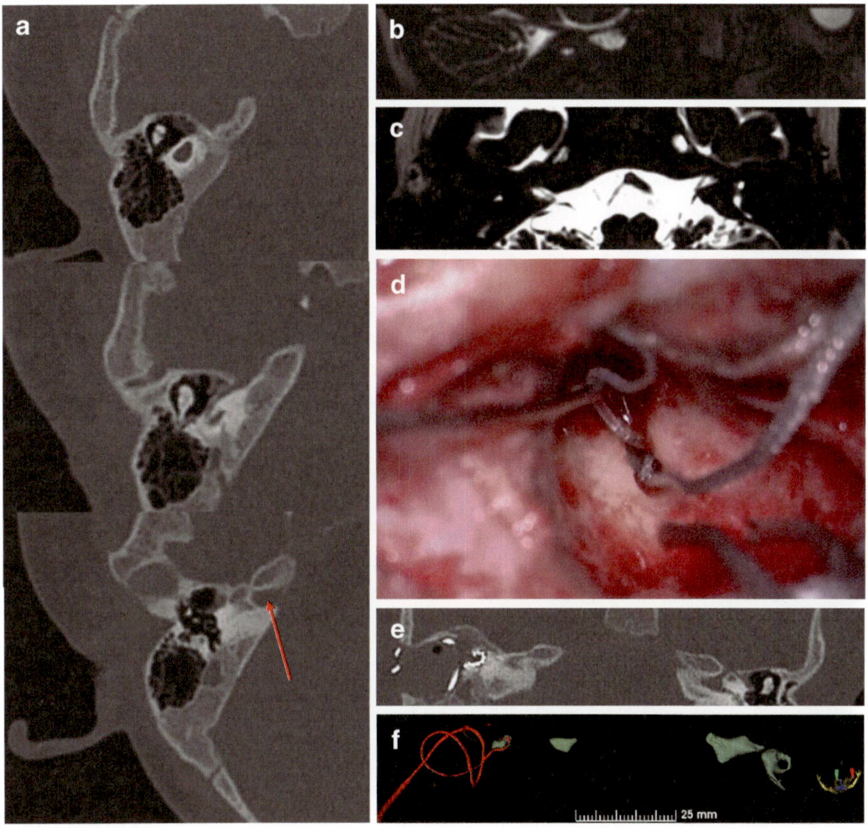

Fig. 6.4 (**a**) The CT of CA shows a narrow slot connecting the otocyst and brain, and the red arrow points to the IAC; (**b**) The oblique sagittal MRI shows that there was no nerve; (**c**) The axial view of MRI; (**d**) The surgical image shows the electrode in the otocyst; (**e**) The postoperative radiological image shows the location of the electrode well; (**f**) The 3D image of the electrode

detect and distinguish all the Ling-6 speech sounds, and the mean disyllabic test score was 53.3%.

6.3.3 Common Cavity Deformity

CCD is a malformation formed by arrested embryonic development at 4 weeks (Jackler et al. 1987) and is defined as the cochlea and vestibule formed into a single, ovoid or round cavity. Theoretically, since there are vestibular and cochlear nerve fibers in the cavity (Sennaroğlu and Bajin 2017), CI is suitable for it. However, because of the uncertainty of the nerve status in the cavity, the outcomes of CCD are varied and usually poor. To overcome the difficulty in CI surgery for CCD, the chief editor of this book developed TLSA combined with a customized electrode (Wei et al. 2017) and has applied this treatment to about 50 patients. The long-term results and programming characteristics have been reported by Zhang et al. (Zhang et al. 2022) and Wei et al. (Wei et al. 2021), and a book focused on CCD that was edited by our team has been published (Li 2022). Inspired by CCD, we have also used this surgical approach for other severe malformations, such as RO and CA (described above), and achieved good results. Because the more severe the malformation, the more likely the encounter with an aberrant facial nerve, TLSA is a good choice to protect the facial nerve. There is an example of treatment for a CCD patient. A two-year-old girl with bilateral CCD and CND underwent CI surgery on her right side with TLSA and a customized electrode (Med-EL, Concerto) (Fig. 6.5a) and the postoperative radiological image showed that the electrode array contacted the cavity wall well (Fig. 6.5b, c). Three years after surgery, her CPA, SIR, MAIS, and MUSS scores were 6, 3, 28, and 16, respectively.

6.3.4 Cochlear Hypoplasia

CH is a better developed IEM than CCD, which has a clear differentiation between the cochlea and vestibule. It can be classified into four types: CH-I, bud-like cochlea; CH-II, cystic hypoplastic cochlea; CH-III, cochlea with less than 2 turns; CI-IV, hypoplastic cochlea (Sennaroğlu and Bajin 2017). CH-I and CH-II are usually accompanied with CND, and since it is usually difficult to expose the round window through the facial recess for these patients, the transcanal approach may be used. In addition, because the cochlea is smaller in cases with CH than in normal ones, thinner and shorter electrodes are advised. In our cases, we also used TLSA for the CH patient. There was a two-year-old girl with CA in her left side and CH in her right side (Fig. 6.6a), and one IAC nerve bundle on each side (Fig. 6.6b, c), so we selected her right side to perform the CI surgery, and TLSA with a small electrode (Med-EL, Sonata) was used for her. Her bud-like cochlea was difficult to expose, and we performed a labyrinthotomy on the canal and inserted the electrode partly into the cochlea (Fig. 6.6d, e). Due to the limited number of electrodes in the cochlea, the outcome was not ideal. After 3 years of surgery, the MAIS score was 4 and the

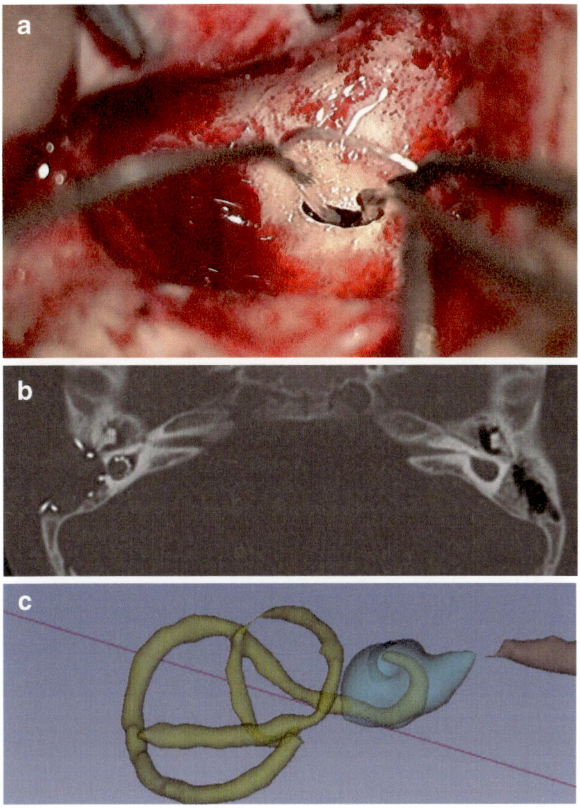

Fig. 6.5 (**a**) The surgical image shows TLSA and the customized electrode used; (**b**). The postoperative radiological image shows the electrode placed well; (**c**) The 3D image of the electrode and cavity

MUSS score was 0. Therefore, some surgeons recommend simultaneous CI and ABI for CH patients between 2 and 3 years of age with barely visible cochlear nerves, and once the CI result was not ideal, the ABI was activated (Freeman and Sennaroglu 2018).

6.3.5 Incomplete Partition Type I

IP-I also has a clear differentiation of the cochlea and vestibule but is featured by a lack of modiolus. The time of developmental arrest of IP-I is similar to that of CH-I, CH-II, and CH-III (Sennaroglu 2016) and is in some cases accompanied with CND. The challenge with CI surgery for IP-I is that cerebrospinal fluid (CSF) gusher is often seen during surgery, and CSF gusher has been reported in about 83% of CI surgery for IP-I cases (Eftekharian et al. 2019). For some patients, CSF leakage occurred even before the surgery, and they were diagnosed with IP-I because of the recurrent meningitis (Chen et al. 2019). For cases with severe CSF gusher, simultaneous repair of the CSF leakage and CI can be done, because if we only repair the CSF leakage first, then the labyrinth may get filled with fibrous tissue

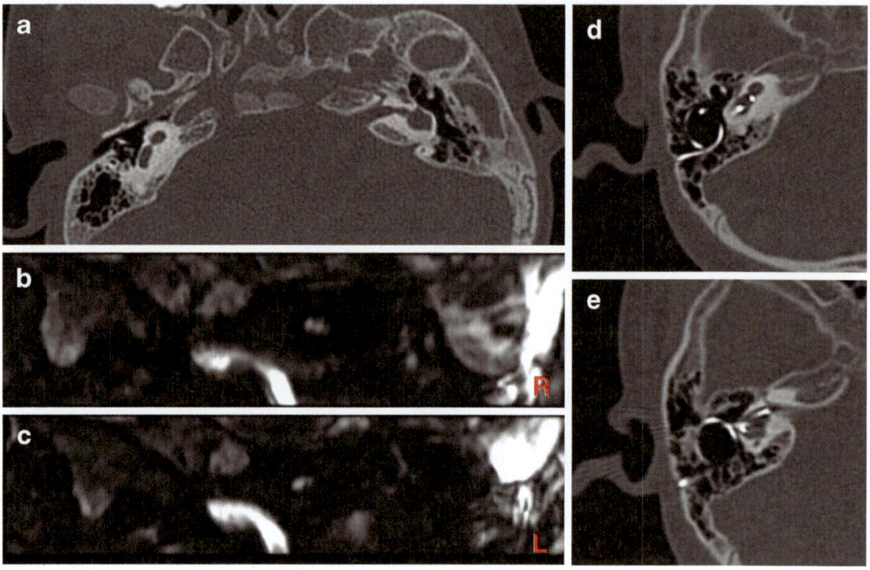

Fig. 6.6 (**a**) The CT shows CH in the right side and CA in the left side; (**b**, **c**) One nerve bundle was present in the IAC on each side; (**d**, **e**) The postoperative electrode array

after some time and CI surgery will become difficult. Short electrodes should be selected for IP-I patients. In our center, we have used the transmastoid lateral semicircular canal approach to repair the CSF leakage and have gone through the round window to implant the cochlea (Chen et al. 2019) for at least five patients, and they all achieved good results with no recurrence of meningitis. For the cases accompanied with CND, some surgeons recommend ABI for them (Sennaroğlu and Bajin 2017), but at our center, we perform CI for the cases that have residual hearing and most of them can achieve sound perception and simple communication. For example, a 10-month-old boy had IP-I in his right side and CA in his left side (Fig. 6.7a), and his right side had a thin cochlear nerve and his left side only had two nerve bundles in the IAC (Fig. 6.7b, c). We selected the right side to implant the cochlea and used a short electrode (Med-EL, Concerto FLEX 15 mm). The postoperative image showed that the electrode was mainly in the basal turn of the cochlea and a few electrodes even turned up into the upper place of the cochlea (Fig. 6.7d, e). The patient's result was good and 3 years after surgery, his CPA, SIR, MAIS, and MUSS scores were 7, 3, 40, and 40, respectively.

6.3.6 Incomplete Partition Type II

IP-II is a common and relatively mild IEM. It is characterized by a defective apical part of the modiolus and is often accompanied with a dilated vestibule and an enlarged vestibular aqueduct. CSF gusher occurs easily even during CI surgery for

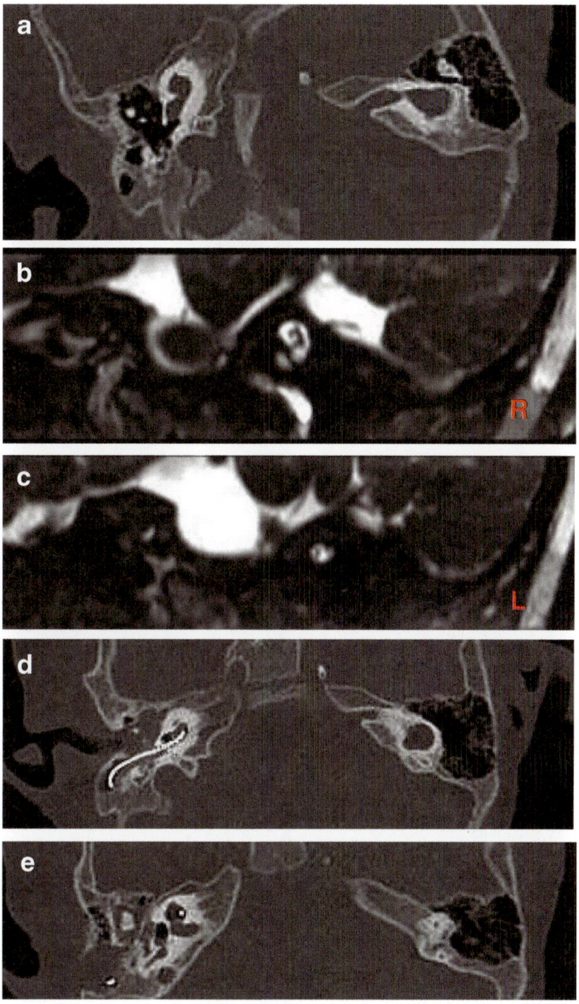

Fig. 6.7 (**a**) The CT shows that the right side has IP-I and the left side has CA; (**b**) The cochlear nerve in the right side was thinner than the facial nerve; (**c**) There were two nerve bundles in the left side; (**d**, **e**) The postoperative electrode in the cochlea

IP-II, but it is not as severe as that during surgery for IP-III and IP-I. An electrode with a silicon stopper is recommended in these cases (Sennaroğlu and Bajin 2017). IP-II is rarely accompanied with CND, in our center there are about 2% CND patients with IP-II. For example, a 5-year-old girl with bilateral IP-II and narrowed IAC (Fig. 6.8a) underwent CI in her right side and the postoperative image showed that the electrode was placed well (Fig. 6.8b, c) in the cochlea. Three years after surgery, her CPA, SIR, MAIS, and MUSS scores were 7, 3, 40, and 32, respectively.

It is worth noting that for bilateral CND patients with bilateral IEM, the side with lighter malformation will be selected as the implant side. For example, if one patient has CCD in one side and CH in the other side, the CH side will be selected for CI (Fig. 6.9). If one side has CCD and the other side has RO, the side with CCD will be selected for CI (Fig. 6.10). If in bilateral IEM patients only one side has CND,

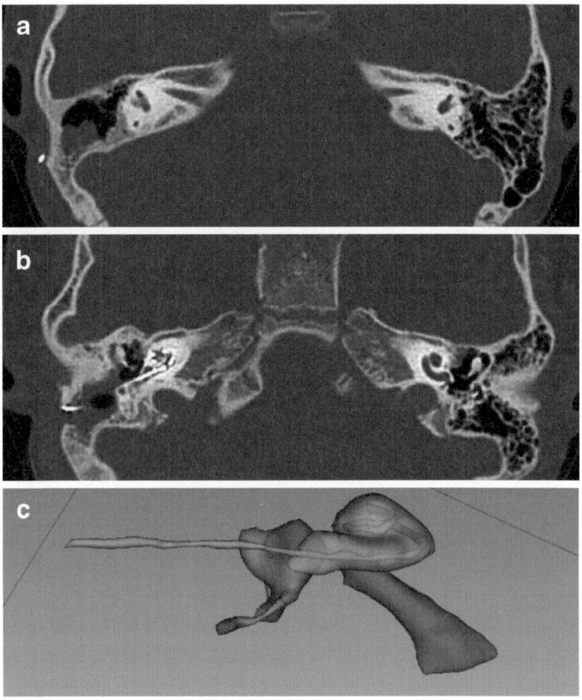

Fig. 6.8 (**a**) The CT shows bilateral narrow IAC; (**b**) The postoperative electrode was placed well; (**c**). The 3D image of electrode

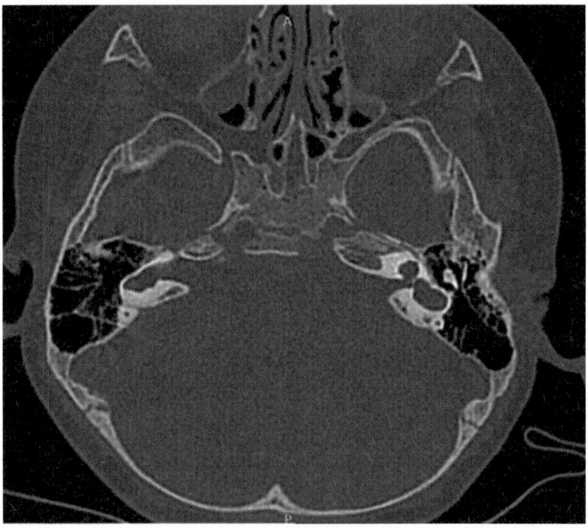

Fig. 6.9 The patient's right side had CCD and the left side had CH, so her left side was selected for CI

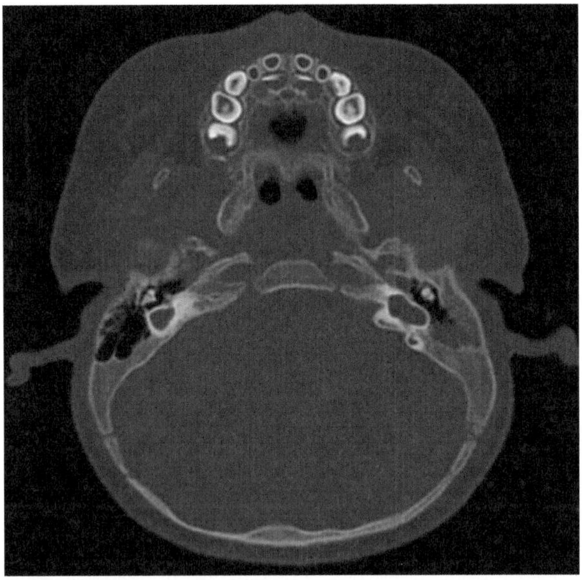

Fig. 6.10 The patient's right side had RO and the left side had CCD, so her left side was selected for CI

then the side without CND will be selected as the implant side. This is because the auditory results of CND are worse than that of single cochlea malformation (Sennaroğlu and Bajin 2017).

6.4 Conclusion

About half the CND patients also have other accompanying IEMs. For the cases without cochlea malformation, we select the side with better cochlear nerve or residual hearing condition for CI. For the cases with cochlear malformation, the side with milder malformation will be selected for CI. The surgical approach and electrode type should be selected according to the classification of the malformation. For some severe malformations, such as CA and CCD, the TLSA and customized electrode can be considered. For some malformations with a small cochlea, a short electrode is preferred. In conclusion, the CI surgery strategies for CND should depend on the patient's individual condition, including the implant age, radiological characteristics, and hearing.

References

Birman CS, Powell HRF, et al. Cochlear implant outcomes in cochlea nerve aplasia and hypoplasia. Otol Neurotol. 2016;37(5):438.

Chen B, Shi Y, et al. Simultaneous repair of cerebrospinal fluid otorrhea and cochlear implantation in two patients with recurrent meningitis and severe inner ear malformation. Int J Pediatr Otorhinolaryngol. 2019;124:147–51.

Coudert A and Van HT, et al. "Vestibular assessment in cochlear implanted children: how to do? When to do? A review of literature." Current Otorhinolaryngology Reports; 2017.

Eftekharian A, Eftekharian K, et al. Cochlear implantation in incomplete partition type I. Eur Arch Otorhinolaryngol. 2019;276(10):2763–8.

Ertugrul G, Aslan F, et al. Children with auditory brainstem implant: how do they perform in motor and language skills? Audiol Neurotol. 2021;26(3):1–9.

Freeman SR, Sennaroglu L. Management of cochlear nerve hypoplasia and aplasia. Adv Otorhinolaryngol. 2018;81:81–92.

Jackler RK, Luxfor WM, et al. Congenital malformations of the inner ear: a classification based on embryogenesis. Laryngoscope. 1987;97:2.

Li Y. Cochlear implantation for common cavity deformity. Springer; 2022.

Morlet T, Pazuniak M, et al. Cochlear nerve deficiency and brain abnormalities in Pediatric patients. Otol Neurotol. 2017;38(3):1.

Orzan E and Pizzamiglio G, et al.. "Correlation of cochlear aperture stenosis with cochlear nerve deficiency in congenital unilateral hearing loss and prognostic relevance for cochlear implantation." Scientific Reports 2021.

Sennaroglu L. "Histopathology of inner ear malformations: do we have enough evidence to explain pathophysiology?" Cochlear Implants International 2016.

Sennaroğlu L, Bajin MD. Classification and current management of inner ear malformations. Balkan Med J. 2017;34(5):397–411.

Shearer AE, Hansen MR. Auditory synaptopathy, auditory neuropathy, and cochlear implantation. Laryngoscope Investig Otolaryngol. 2019;4:429.

Wei X, Li Y, et al. Predicting auditory outcomes from radiological imaging in cochlear implant patients with cochlear nerve deficiency. Otol Neurotol. 2017;38:5.

Wei X, Zhang H, et al. Application of multiplanar volume reconstruction technique for the assessment of electrode location and analysis of the correlation to Cochlear programming and performance in common cavity deformity. Front Neurol. 2021;12:783225.

Wei and Xingmei, et al. Slotted Labyrinthotomy approach with customized electrode for patients with common cavity deformity. The Laryngoscope: A Medical Journal for Clinical and Research Contributions in Otolaryngology, Head and Neck Medicine and Surgery, Facial Plastic and Reconstructive Surgery 2018.

Zhang L, Chen B, et al. Analysis of long-term cochlear implantation outcomes and correlation with imaging characteristics in patients with common cavity deformity. Front Neurosci. 2022;16:857855.

7 Programming Cochlear Implants for Cochlear Nerve Deficiency

Ying Kong, Xingmei Wei, Shujin Xue, Jingyuan Chen, and Simeng Lu

Cochlear implant programming, an important postoperative procedure to obtain hearing rehabilitation effectively, contains initial stimulation and follow-up programming. Initial stimulation is the first programming after surgery. The audiologist installs an external device and programs the cochlear implant system for recipients, which allows the recipients to receive sound (Pires et al. 2018). The aim of initial stimulation is letting the patient adapt to the device and provide the patient with a detectable and comfortable sound. The patient can then begin adaptive auditory and speech training and rehabilitation. Array position and the number of electrodes located in the cochlea must be clarified through postoperative radiological images before initial stimulation. Meanwhile, intraoperative monitoring outcomes should be acquired, including intraoperative impedance, electrically evoked compound action potentials (ECAP), and electrically evoked auditory brainstem responses, to confirm the implant's integrity and determine the entire auditory pathway's function (Wieringen et al. 2008).

Y. Kong (✉) · X. Wei · S. Xue · J. Chen · S. Lu
Key Laboratory of Otolaryngology Head and Neck Surgery (Capital Medical University), Ministry of Education, Beijing, China

Department of Otorhinolaryngology Head and Neck Surgery, Beijing Tongren Hospital, Capital Medical University, Beijing, China

Y. Li (ed.), *Cochlear Implantation for Cochlear Nerve Deficiency*,
https://doi.org/10.1007/978-981-19-5892-2_7

7.1 Initial Stimulation

1. Electrode impedances are measured first during initial stimulation. Electrode impedances are mainly used to measure the electrode function in the cochlea, and electrodes with abnormal electrode impedance (open or short) should be closed.
2. To select sound processing strategy and stimulus parameters: Generally, the default parameters from the software are selected, which include sound processing strategy, stimulation mode, stimulation rate, pulse width (PW), and number of stimulation electrodes.
3. Threshold levels measurement

   The threshold levels (T levels) are the softest electrical input levels detectable by the user for each electrode contact (Goehring et al. 2014).

   The measurement method varies according to patients' age. Adults, adolescents, or older children can use pure tone audiometry. Children can use pediatric behavior audiometry, such as visual reinforcement audiometry (VRA) and conditioned play audiometry (CPA).
4. Upper-Stimulation Levels Measurement

   The definitions of upper stimulus levels of different manufacturers are different (Wolfe and Schafer 2014). In the Nucleus system, the upper-stimulation levels are called comfortable levels (C levels). In the MED-EL system, the upper-stimulation levels are called the "maximum comfort level" (MCL). In the Advanced Bionics system, it is called the "most comfortable" (M-level).

   During programming, the loudness discomfort threshold (LDL) of a specific electrode is gradually reached and the comfort threshold can be set to the stimulation intensity below the LDL.
5. Create optimized MAP.

   After the above tests are performed, go live to allow the patient to listen to environmental sounds and speech sounds to ensure the audibility and comfort of the sound, which can be assessed by Ling's six sound test or speech test.

   After the initial stimulation, it is necessary to explain the usage and caution the patients and their families, as well as explain the methods to observe patients' response to sounds, in order to provide feedbacks and follow-up programming.

7.2 Follow-Up Programming

Follow-up programming is usually arranged at 1 month, 3 months, 6 months, 9 months, and 12 months after the initial stimulation. With the use time of cochlear implantation (CI) and the stabilization of MAP, the programming interval can be gradually extended to either half a year or one year. The purpose of follow-up programming is mainly to detect the device and adjust the parameters, as well as to consult, evaluate, and solve the patient's listening problems, so as to ensure the best auditory performance of the patient is maintained. During follow-up programming, the contents are mainly the same as those for initial stimulation, sometimes the coding strategy and stimulation parameters need to be changed according to the patients' feedback, impedance results, and overall evaluation results. Based on the cooperating ability of the patient, the loudness balancing test and pitch scaling can be added during programming to optimize the auditory outcomes.

For infants and young children or patients with multiple disabilities who cannot cooperate with behavioral tests, the upper-stimulation level or threshold can also be estimated based on objective tests. In clinical practice, the electrically evoked stapedius reflex threshold is used (Wolfe et al. 2017; Jace et al. 2018; Kosaner et al. 2018). In addition, the threshold and upper-stimulation level can be estimated by electrically ECAP (Yamazaki et al. 2015; De Vos et al. 2017; Kosaner et al. 2018). Although these objective tests in early programming can provide the patient with an audible and comfortable sound, it may not be in the best condition. With the continuous input of sounds and the development of auditory behaviors, it is still necessary to conduct accurate behavioral audiometry as early as possible, which are still the most basic and effective test technique to determine the best settings for CI (Young et al. 2012).

The threshold levels and upper-stimulation levels should be measured as accurately as possible. If the T levels are set too low, the patient may not hear sounds with low loudness. If the T levels are set too high, the patient may experience greater environmental noise and limited electrical dynamic range. Low setting of upper-stimulation levels may have a negative impact on speech recognition, voice quality, and the ability to monitor the patient's own voice. If the settings are too high, it may cause discomfort to the sound and further lead to patient conflict with the device, and affect the speech recognition and sound quality.

7.3 Tips for Programming of Cochlear Nerve Deficiency

The content and steps of programming for patients with CND are the same as those for other patients. However, since the inner ear structure of CND patients can be normal or deformed, there are some points that are different from other patients and require attention during programming. The number of electrodes located in the cochlea must be clarified through postoperative images before initial stimulation, especially in patients with inner ear malformation, and the extracochlear electrodes need to be turned off. Since patients with CND have fewer remaining auditory nerves and worse neural synchronization, they require higher intensity of electrical stimulation (Young et al. 2012). When measuring upper-stimulation levels, if the patient cannot acquire a satisfactory loudness level even with the maximum stimulation current, the PW can be appropriately increased. The deformed cochlea or abnormally routed facial nerve in patients with inner ear malformations (Wu et al. 2015) may cause facial nerve stimulation symptoms such as twitching of the lower eyelid and the corners of the mouth and eyes, face twitch, and other symptoms during the measurement of MCL. Reducing the stimulation current, increasing the PW, changing to triphasic pulse stimulation, or closing the active electrode can be chosen according to the different devices to relieve the symptoms of facial nerve stimulation (Karuna et al. 2019). For some CND patients with accompanying CCD, when some electrodes are stimulated, vestibular nerve stimulation symptoms such as leaning forward or tilting back and forth will be displayed (Wei et al. 2021). Therefore, paying close attention to the subtle reactions of patients while programming is necessary.

Many studies about CND have shown that for CND patients, a slower stimulation rate can help them obtain more benefits from CI (Peterson et al. 2003; Teagle et al. 2010; Pelosi et al. 2012). He et al. (He et al. 2018) found that the absolute refractory period of the cochlear nerve was longer in CND patients than in non-CND patients, and a prolonged absolute refractory period was associated with a decreased number of auditory nerve fibers and poor function of cochlear nerve, which can partially explain the rationale for using a slower stimulation rate in CND patients. Since the function of the cochlear nerve varies greatly among individual CND patients, the default stimulation rate is used in initial programming, and the simulation rate is then adjusted based on feedback and overall evaluation.

The study of postoperative ECAP of CND patients (He et al. 2018) found that the rate used to elicit ECAP varies with the location of electrodes, and as the stimulation moved from the basal turn to the apical turn of the cochlea, the rate used to elicit ECAP gradually decreased, indicating that the number of auditory nerves decreased from the basal turn to the apical turn of the cochlea. Miller et al. (Miller et al. 2000) found that the presence of the ECAP depends on the availability of sufficient cochlear nerve fibers responding synchronously to electrical stimulation. During the programming, we also found that the CND patients responded better to high-frequency than to low-frequency, and the low-frequency region required a higher stimulation current than the high-frequency region. Patients are also more sensitive to high-frequency sounds than low-frequency sounds in the initial postoperative auditory and speech rehabilitation. These results demonstrate that patients with CND have fewer cochlear nerve fibers in the low-frequency region than in the high-frequency region, and have better neural survival at the base turn than at the apex of the cochlea. Thus, CND patients showed better function of the cochlear nerve in the high-frequency region than in the low-frequency region.

Since the overall postoperative auditory and speech rehabilitation outcome of CND patients is worse than that of patients with normal cochlear nerves, it is very important for the audiologist to communicate with CND patients or their families and establish proper expectations. After each follow-up programming, the audiologist should discuss with the patient and families, summarize the progress or changes after the last follow-up, and point out problems and difficulties which still exist, in order to set up new goals, make plans for the next period, and help them establish reasonable expectations. For CND patients, the programming interval is also recommended to be shorter than that for other patients, in order that we can follow up and adjust parameters dynamically and obtain the patient's MAP changes and rehabilitation efficacy in time.

7.4 Our Cases and Experience

7.4.1 Special Cases

We will share a case who achieved good results after adjusting the programming parameters and further demonstrate the importance of appropriate programming for CND patient. A boy was referred following failed the newborn hearing screening, and he was diagnosed with bilateral cochlear nerve dysplasia and no cochlear malformation. The patient presented with overall growth retardation combined with callosal agenesis. At 4 months old, hearing aids are used alternately on both sides, and his parents can observe his responses to loud sounds. The patient underwent left cochlear implantation at the age of 9 months, and continued to use hearing aids on the right side. The COCHLEAR CI512 electrode was used, and the postoperative radiology images showed that the electrodes were all located in the cochlea. Electrodes impedances were all normal when initial stimulation. The stimulation pulse width was 50s and stimulation rate was 500 pulses per second (pps) (Fig. 7.1). The child was not sensitive to sound, just testing No.10 electrode we can observe him turning head to find sound. When using the automatic NRT test, the electrodes No. 1, 11, 16, and 22 did not elicit a clear waveform (Fig. 7.2). Then we adjusted the MAP and GO LIVE, when clapping hands loudly we observed the child's eyes raising. We advised his parents to help the child perform auditory rehabilitation and observe the child's responses to various sounds.

During the second follow-up programming, the parents replied that the child was willing to using the cochlear implant device, and they observed the child had awareness to moderate-intensity sounds of drums, piano, cymbals, and the voice "a, i, m".

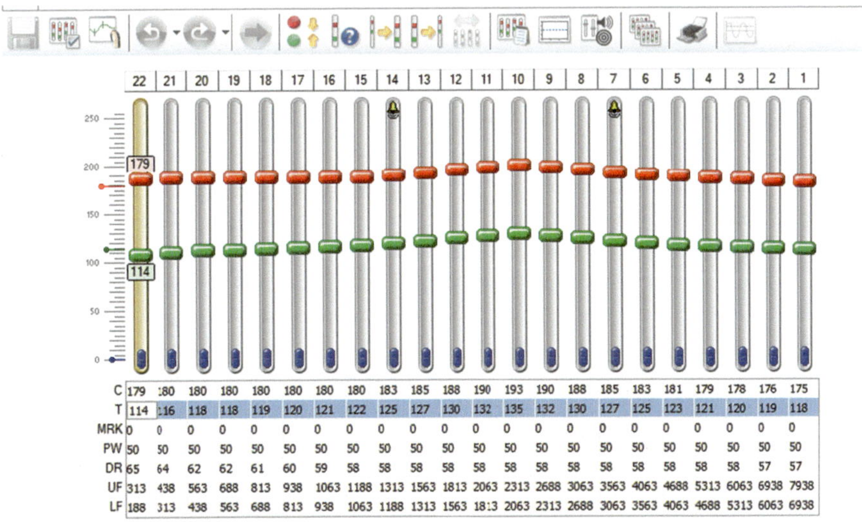

Fig. 7.1 The initial stimulation MAP

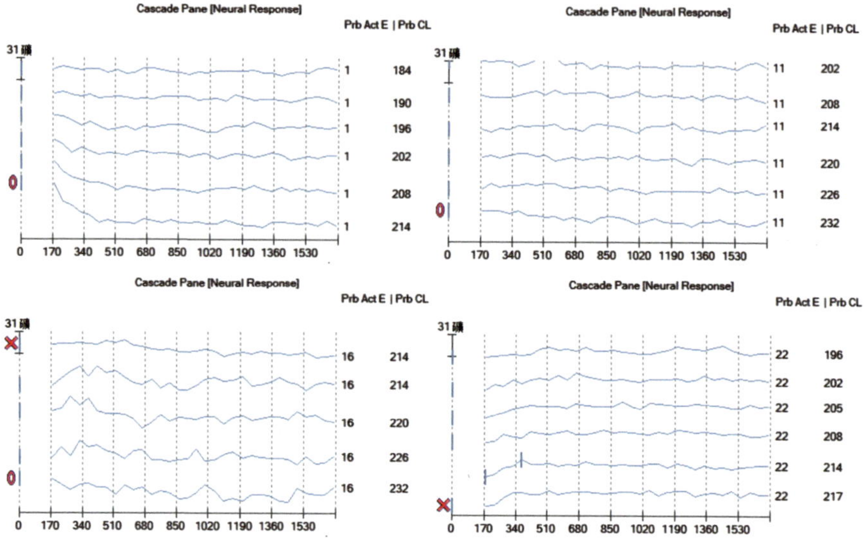

Fig. 7.2 The automatic NRT outcome (NRT could not be elicited on electrodes No. 1, 11, 16, and 22)

When we adjusted NRT with manual parameters (Probe pulse width; Probe rate; Gain; Number of sweeps; Recording electrode active), clear waveform can be elicited on no.3, 6, 9, 12, 15, 21 electrodes, and each waveform is well differentiated (Fig. 7.3). The MAP was readjusted according to the NRT threshold and the child's acoustic outcomes (Fig. 7.4).

Because of the dysplasia of the corpus callosum, the child's general development is delayed. His parents continued to help him carry out auditory and speech training as well as physical movement rehabilitation. During each follow-up programming, we communicated with his parents to summarize the child's progress and set up new goals for the next period. The child is making continuous slow progress. At 6 months after initial stimulation, the child's response to environmental and speech sounds increased significantly, and he also responded well to his name. At the same time, his self-pronunciation increased, and the pronunciation began to have a tone.

As the child's response and sensitivity to sound increases, the MAP can be fine-adjusted after the VRA test can be performed (Fig. 7.5). At present, the child has been used CI for 2 years, and the average aided threshold on the CI side is 31.5dBHL. The auditory speech questionnaire evaluation results were IT-MAIS = 6, MUSS = 2, CAP = 2, SIR = 1. Because the child has comorbidities, the score is lower than the average level of the children in the CND group of our center, but the parents are very satisfied with the progress the child has made so far.

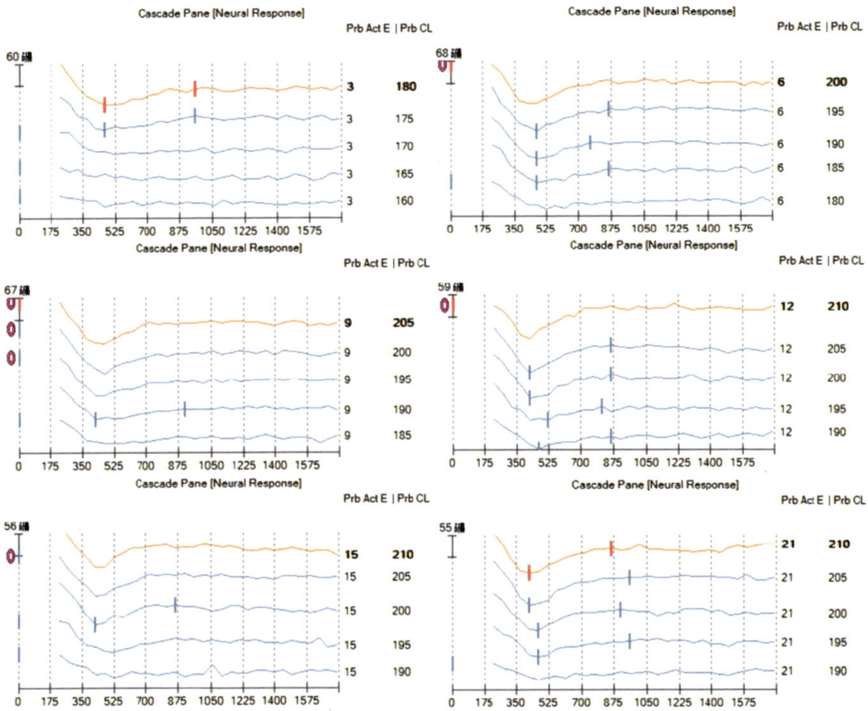

Fig. 7.3 The NRT test with manual adjusted parameters (NRT could be elicited on electrodes No. 3, 6, 9, 12, 15, and 21)

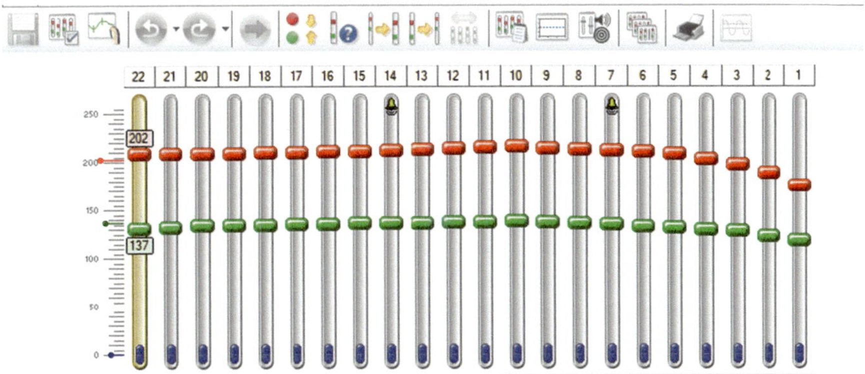

C	202	202	201	202	203	203	204	204	205	206	207	208	209	207	206	205	204	202	196	190	182	168
T	137	138	140	140	140	141	141	142	142	143	144	144	145	144	142	141	139	138	136	135	129	125
MRK	0	0	0	0	0	0	0	0	0	C	0	0	0	0	0	0	0	0	0	0	0	0
PW	50	50	50	50	50	50	50	50	50	50	50	50	50	50	50	50	50	50	50	50	50	50
DR	65	64	61	62	63	62	63	62	63	63	63	64	64	63	64	64	65	64	60	55	53	43
UF	313	438	563	688	813	938	1063	1188	1313	1563	1813	2063	2313	2688	3063	3563	4063	4688	5313	6063	6938	7938
LF	188	313	438	563	688	813	938	1063	1188	1313	1563	1813	2063	2313	2688	3063	3563	4063	4688	5313	6063	6938

Fig. 7.4 The second programming MAP according to NRT test outcomes

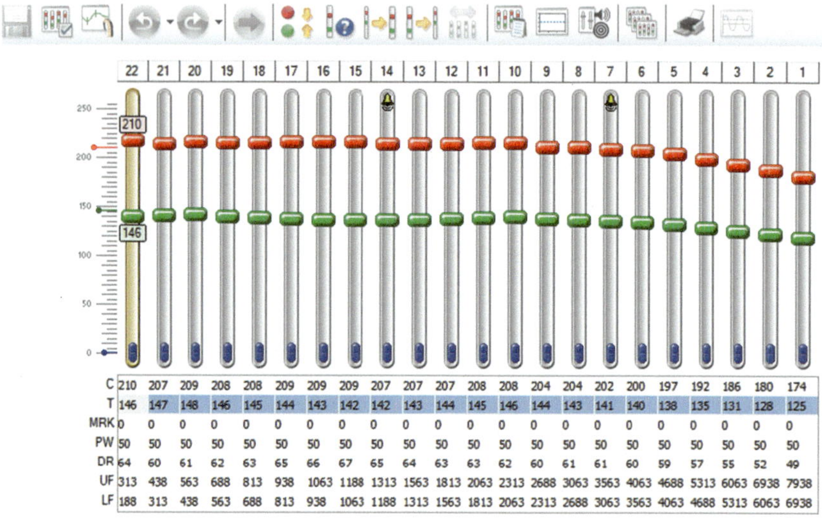

Fig. 7.5 The fine-adjusted MAP, and VRA can be performed

7.4.2 Cases Series and Statistical Results

Our center has rich experience with programming of CND patients, because the number of CND cases in our CI center is one of the largest in China. Ninety CND patients and seventy-nine normal patients (as the control group) who underwent CI surgery at our center from June 2007 to June 2020 were included in this study. We collected the programming parameters one year after surgery and collected the outcomes measured by categories of auditory performance (CAP), speech intelligibility rating (SIR), meaningful auditory integration scale (for age 3–6 year)/infant-toddler (for<3 years of age) meaningful auditory integration scale (MAIS/IT-MAIS), and meaningful use of speech scale (MUSS) two years after surgery. These patients were all under 6 years of age when the device was implanted. In the CND group, we further divided patients into the normal CND group without cochlear malformation and the malformed group with cochlear malformation. Each group was divided into Med-EL and Cochlear groups according to their device manufactures for the convenience of comparison. The number of cases, sex, side, implanted age, implant, processor, coding strategy, stimulation rate, pulse characteristics, and PW are listed in Table 7.1. We then compared the impedances, stimulation level, and outcomes among these groups.

As shown in Table 7.1, for the Med-EL device, while the coding strategies of the normal CND and normal groups were mainly FS4, a few cases used fine structure processing (FSP) and continuous interleaved sampling (CIS), and for the malformed CND group, FS4-p and high-definition continuous interleaved sampling (HDCIS), except for CIS, FS4, and FSP, were also applied in some cases. HDCIS is mainly used for patients with severe inner malformation, such as CCD. The reason may be

Table 7.1 The patients' grouping, basic information, and programming parameters

		Med-EL			Cochlear		
		Normal CND	Malformed CND	Normal	Normal CND	Malformed CND	Normal
Sample number		22 (24 ears)	42 (45 ears)	49 (52 ears)	15	11	29
Gender	M	10	19	32	6	6	18
	F	12	23	17	9	5	11
Side	R	8	19	11	7	3	4
	L	12	20	35	8	8	25
	Bilateral	2	3	3	0	0	0
Implanted age M (min, max)		1.46 (1–6)	1.42 (0–6)	1 (0.5–6)	2.17 (1.08–5.75)	2.33 (0–5)	3.0 (0.92–6)
Implant		C40+ 1 Mix10xx 11 Sonata 12	C40+ 1 Mix10xx 30 Sonata 14	Mi10xx 15 PULSAR 13 Sonata 24	CI24R(CA) 3 CI512 4 CI522 4 CI24RE(CA) 3 CI24RE(ST) 1	CI24R(CA) 2 CI24R(ST) 1 CI422 1 CI512 1 CI522 2 CI24RE(ST) 4	CI24R(CA) 29 CI24RE(CA) 3
Processor		OPUS1 9; OPUS2 13 Sonnet 1 TEMOPO+ 1	OPUS1 13 OPUS2 30 Round2 1 TEMOPO+ 1	OPUS1 19 OPUS 2 33	CP802 4 CP810 4 CP900 series 3 Freedom 3 Sprint 2	CP802 6 CP900 series 2 Freedom 1 Sprint 2	ESPrit 3G10 Freedom 10 Sprint 9

(continued)

Table 7.1 (continued)

	Med-EL			Cochlear		
	Normal CND	Malformed CND	Normal	Normal CND	Malformed CND	Normal
Coding strategy	CIS 1 FS4 20 FSP 3	CIS 1 FS4 38 FS4-p 1 HDCIS 5	CIS 1 FS4 41 FSP 10	ACE 15	ACE 11	ACE 29
Stimulation rate	Reduced 5 Maximal 19	Reduced 2 Maximal 43	Reduced 39 Maximal 13	250pps 1 500pps 1 720pps 1 900pps 12	720pps 1 900pps 10	900pps 29
Pulse characteristics	Triphasic 1 Biphasic 21	Triphasic 1 Biphasic 44	Biphasic 51			
Pulse width				25 μs 9 37 μs 2 50 μs 1 100 μs 1 200 μs 1	25 μs 7 37 μs 2 50 μs 2	25 μs 29

that limited spiral ganglion affects their receiving of more sound information, which is a reminder that if the patient's response to the default strategy is poor during programming of the malformed case, more strategies could be tried. For the Cochlear device, they all used Advanced Combination Encoder strategies. In the Cochlear group, the stimulation rate of the normal group was all 900 pps. However, some CND patients used a lower stimulation rate, such as 750, 500, and 720 pps, which is consistent with other reports. The reason for this is that a reduced stimulation rate can help the cochlear nerve synchronization better because the absolute refractory period of cochlear nerve in CND patients is prolonged (He et al. 2018). However, for the Med-EL group, there were 39 cases (76%) that used reduced rates in the normal group, this is because the majority of patients in this group underwent CI in 2010, which was when the first version of FS4 was released and the stimulation rates were reduced to 750 pps for reducing the masking of temporal information. Higher stimulation rates (up to 1600 pps) were available when the software was updated later in 2015 (Riss et al. 2014). In the Med-EL group, two patients in the CND group used triphasic pulses and the other patients all used biphasic pulses. The use of triphasic pulse can reduce the neurogenic stimulation, and further reduce the facial stimulation (Braun et al. 2019). Facial nerve stimulation occurred for two patients using triphasic pulses, and the symptoms were relieved after adjusting the parameters. The PW of the Cochlear device can be adjusted. For normal patients, 25 μs is used, and in CND groups, other higher PWs such as 37, 50, 100, and 200 μs are used in a few patients. This also demonstrates that increased PW is sometimes necessary to increase the stimuli efficiency for CND patients (He et al. 2020).

The average impedance, stimulation level, and outcomes of the Med-EL and Cochlear groups are listed in Tables 7.2 and 7.3. The above data for normal CND, malformed CND, and normal groups were compared for each device group by the *Kruskal Wallis test*. The impedance was not different in each group of the Med-EL group. The MCL of the CND group was significantly higher than that of the normal group ($p < 0.05$), the CAP, SIR, MAIS/IT-MAIS, and MUSS scores of the normal group were significantly better than that of the CND group ($p < 0.05$), but the MCL and questionnaires for the normal CND and malformed CND groups had no

Table 7.2 The median and range of average impedance, maximum comfort level, and outcomes of the Med-EL group

	Average impedance (kΩ)	Average MCL (qu)	CAP	SIR	MAIS/ IT-MAIS	MUSS
Normal CND (M (min, max))	6.94 (3.78, 10.32)	21.38 (9.73, 39.970)	4 (1,7)	2 (1,5)	29 (9,40)	8 (1,35)
Malformed CND (M (min, max))	7.25 (2.92,12.68)	23.36 (10.91, 45.28)	5 (1,6)	2 (1,4)	30 (4,40)	12 (0, 33)
Normal (M (min, max))	7.03 (5.01,10.41)	15.31 (7.52, 22.18)	6 (3,7)	4 (1,5)	35 (13,40)	27 (1,40)

CND cochlear nerve deficiency, *MCL* maximum comfort level, *M* medium, *min* minimum, *max* maximum

Table 7.3 The median and range of average impedance of four modes, T and C levels, and outcomes of the Cochlear group

		CG (kΩ)	MP1 (kΩ)	MP2 (kΩ)	MP1 + 2 (kΩ)	C*PW (CL)	T*PW (CL)	CAP	SIR	MAIS/ IT-MAIs	MUSS
Normal CND	Medium	9.4955	11.8677	10.8250	10.8873	5384.0909	3755.6818	5.0000	2.0000	24.0000	8.0000
	Minimum	4.37	9.03	7.06	6.74	3754.55	2707.95	1.00	1.00	4.00	0.00
	Maximum	14.25	16.81	15.88	15.81	32745.45	27354.55	7.00	5.00	34.00	38.00
Malformed CND	Medium	6.7500	8.2682	8.0300	7.9041	4928.4091	4360.2273	4.0000	2.0000	26.0000	15.0000
	Minimum	4.36	6.56	6.04	5.58	4063.64	3089.77	2.00	1.00	14.00	2.00
	Maximum	10.97	10.44	10.77	8.67	9593.18	7084.09	5.00	2.00	34.00	24.00
Normal	Medium	8.1245	10.9159	9.9032	9.5223	4192.0455	3290.9091	6.0000	4.0000	38.0000	30.0000
	Minimum	4.90	7.18	6.53	6.06	3370.45	2620.45	5.00	2.00	24.00	10.00
	Maximum	13.59	18.45	14.77	74.73	5843.18	4418.18	7.00	5.00	40.00	40.00

C C level, *T* T level, *CL* current level, *PW* pulse width, *CND* cochlear nerve deficiency difference ($p > 0.05$). For the Cochlear group, the four types of impedances of the malformed CND group were significantly lower than that of the normal CND and normal group ($p < 0.05$). This difference may be because the malformed CND group mainly used straight electrode array, whose impedance is usually lower than that of the contour electrode. It can be explained that the straight array is mainly surrounded by conductive fluid, while the "modiolus-hugging" contour electrode is close to bone, causing more fibrous tissue to develop and increasing the impedance (Wermeskerken et al. 2006). The T level, C level, and outcomes of the Cochlear group are similar to those of the Med-EL group, and stimulus level of the CND group is higher but the questionnaire scores are lower than that of the normal group ($p < 0.05$), and the normal CND and malformed group had no difference. Other studies also found that the stimulus of the CND group was higher, and the reason for this was that the few CN fibers and poor function in CND require higher electrical charge per unit phase to achieve auditory perception (Teagle et al. 2010; Buchman et al. 2011). The normal CND and malformed CND had no difference, maybe because the main influence factor of stimulus is CN function but not inner ear structure. Many studies have confirmed that CND patients have poorer outcomes than normal patients (Yamazaki et al. 2015; Wei et al. 2017). There were different conclusions regarding the influence of inner ear malformation on the outcomes, while some studies found that there was no difference in the outcome of different types of anomalies (Michael et al. 2012; Daneshi et al. 2020), others found that the more severe the malformation, the worse the results (Shi et al. 2019). The different conclusions may be related to the sample size and involved malformations. To the best of our knowledge, there was no study comparing the outcomes of CND combined with inner ear malformation, and we found no outcome difference between normal and malformed cochleas, maybe because CND is the main factor affecting the outcome (Farhood et al. 2017).

In addition, there were 12 (7%) cases in our study where non-auditory responses, such as face twitch or tilting forth and back, occurred, and all the cases were in the CND group, among which 8 were in malformed group. Another report also found that the non-auditory response usually occurred in patients with malformations, especially in those with CCD (Ahmad and Lokman 2005).

7.5 Conclusion

The programming for CND patients has its particular challenges, so the audiologist should be careful while programming CND cases. The stimulation level for CND is usually higher than that for non-CND ones, and in some cases, a lower stimulation rate and higher PW can be selected for better results. In severe malformed CND cases, non-auditory responses such as facial nerve stimulation may occur. Reducing the stimulation current, increasing the PW, changing to triphasic pulses stimulation, or closing the active electrode can be done to relieve the symptoms. Though the outcomes of CND patients are usually poorer than that of normal patients, optimized programming strategy should be explored for them to achieve better reception.

References

Ahmad RL, Lokman S. Cochlear implantation in congenital cochlear abnormalities. Med J Malays. 2005;60(3):379.

Braun K, Walker K, et al. Triphasic pulses in cochlear implant patients with facial nerve stimulation. Otol Neurotol. 2019;40(10):1.

Buchman CA, Teagle H, et al. Cochlear implantation in children with labyrinthine anomalies and cochlear nerve deficiency: implications for auditory brainstem implantation. Laryngoscope. 2011;121(9):1979–88.

Daneshi A, Farhadi M, et al. Cochlear implantation in children with inner ear malformation: a multicenter study on auditory performance and speech production outcomes. Int J Pediatr Otorhinolaryngol. 2020;132:109901.

De Vos JJ, Biesheuvel JD, et al. Use of electrically evoked compound action potentials for Cochlear implant fitting. Ear Hear. 2017;1

Farhood Z, Nguyen SA, et al. Cochlear implantation in inner ear malformations: systematic review of speech perception outcomes and intraoperative findings. Otolaryngol Head Neck Surg. 2017;156(3):194599817696502.

Goehring JL, Neff DL, et al. Pitch ranking, electrode discrimination, and physiological spread of excitation using current steering in cochlear implants. J Acoust Soc Am. 2014;136(6):3159–71.

He S, Shahsavarani BS, et al. Responsiveness of the electrically stimulated cochlear nerve in children with cochlear nerve deficiency. Ear Hear. 2018;1

He S, Xu L, et al. Effect of increasing pulse phase duration on neural responsiveness of the electrically stimulated cochlear nerve. Ear Hear. 2020;6:1. Publish Ahead of Print

Jace W, Rene G, et al. Measurement of the electrically evoked stapedial reflex response with wideband acoustic reflectance measurement. J Am Acad Audiol. 2018;29(4):337–47.

Karuna, et al. Imaging of pediatric hearing loss. Neuroimaging Clin N Am. 2019;29(1):103–15.

Kosaner J, Spitzer P, et al. Comparing eSRT and eCAP measurements in pediatric MED-EL cochlear implant users. Cochlear Implants Int. 2018;1

Michael and Pakdaman, et al. Cochlear implantation in children with anomalous cochleovestibular anatomy. Otolaryngol Head Neck Surg: Official Journal of American Academy of Otolaryngology-Head and Neck Surgery. 2012.

Miller CA, Abbas PJ, et al. An improved method of reducing stimulus artifact in the electrically evoked whole-nerve potential. Ear Hear. 2000;21(4):280–90.

Pelosi S, Rivas A, et al. Stimulation rate reduction and auditory development in poorly performing cochlear implant users with auditory neuropathy. Otol Neurotol. 2012;33(9):1502–6.

Peterson A, Shallop J, et al. Outcomes of cochlear implantation in children with auditory neuropathy. J Am Acad Audiol. 2003;14(4):188–201.

Pires JS, Melo AS, et al. Facial nerve stimulation after cochlear implantation: our experience in 448 adult patients. Cochlear Implants Int. 2018;1

Riss D, Hamzavi JS, et al. FS4, FS4-P, and FSP: a 4-month crossover study of three fine structure sound-coding strategies. Ear Hear. 2014;35:6.

Shi Y, Li Y, et al. Cochlear implants for patients with inner ear malformation: experience in a cohort of 877 surgeries. Clin Otolaryngol. 2019;44:4.

Teagle H, Roush PA, et al. Cochlear implantation in children with auditory neuropathy Spectrum disorder. Ear Hear. 2010;31(3):325–35.

Wei X, Li Y, et al. Predicting auditory outcomes from radiological imaging in Cochlear implant patients with Cochlear nerve deficiency. Otol Neurotol. 2017;38:5.

Wei X, Zhang H, et al. Application of multiplanar volume reconstruction technique for the assessment of electrode location and analysis of the correlation to cochlear programming and performance in common cavity deformity. Front Neurol. 2021;12:783225.

Wermeskerken G, Olphen A, et al. Intra- and postoperative electrode impedance of the straight and contour arrays of the nucleus 24 cochlear implant: relation to T and C levels. Int J Audiol. 2006;45(9):537–44.

Wieringen AV, Macherey O, et al. Alternative pulse shapes in electrical hearing. Hear Res. 2008;242(1–2):154–63.

Wolfe J, Gilbert M, et al. Optimizations for the electrically-evoked stapedial reflex threshold measurement in Cochlear implant recipients. Ear Hearing. 2017;38(2):255.

Wolfe and Schafer. Programming cochlear implants, Programming Cochlear Implants. 2014.

Wu CM, Lee LA, et al. Impact of cochlear nerve deficiency determined using 3-dimensional magnetic resonance imaging on hearing outcome in children with cochlear implants. Otol Neurotol. 2015;36(1):1.

Yamazaki H, Leigh J, et al. Usefulness of MRI and EABR testing for predicting CI outcomes immediately after cochlear implantation in cases with cochlear nerve deficiency. Otol Neurotol. 2015;36:977.

Young NM, Kim FM, et al. Pediatric cochlear implantation of children with eighth nerve deficiency. Int J Pediatr Otorhinolaryngol. 2012;76:10.

Cochlear Implantation Outcomes of Cochlear Nerve Deficiency

8

Simeng Lu, Xingmei Wei, Ying Kong, Biao Chen, Lifang Zhang, Shujin Xue, Mengge Yang, Xinyue Zou, Xinyi Zhang, and Yongxin Li

8.1 Auditory and Speech Outcomes of Cochlear Nerve Deficiency (CND)

Studies on auditory and speech outcomes after (cochlear implantation) CI in patients with CND showed that patients could benefit from CI, but outcomes vary greatly (Wu et al. 2015; Wei et al. 2017; Freeman and Sennaroglu 2018). In general, patients with CND have worse postoperative CI outcomes than those without CND, and some patients do not benefit from CI at all (Wei et al. 2017; Yousef et al. 2021).

8.1.1 Assessment

Depending on the patient's ability, previous literature has used mainly questionnaire results. Hearing performance is often assessed using the Categorical Auditory Performance (CAP) and the Infant-Toddler Meaningful Auditory Integration Scale (IT-MAIS) or MAIS scores. The CAP is an 8-point scale ranging from 0 (no awareness of environmental sounds) to 7 (use of a telephone with a known listener).

S. Lu · X. Wei · Y. Kong · B. Chen · L. Zhang · S. Xue · M. Yang · X. Zou · X. Zhang · Y. Li (✉)
Department of Otorhinolaryngology Head and Neck Surgery, Beijing Tongren Hospital, Capital Medical University, Beijing, China

Key Laboratory of Otolaryngology Head and Neck Surgery (Capital Medical University), Ministry of Education, Beijing, China

Y. Li (ed.), *Cochlear Implantation for Cochlear Nerve Deficiency*,
https://doi.org/10.1007/978-981-19-5892-2_8

IT-MAIS/MAIS (IT-MAIS for patients aged <3 years and MAIS for patients aged >3 years) is scored on a scale of 0–40 and is used to assess auditory performance, including vocal variation, self-articulation, and the ability to understand the meaning of sounds.

Speech outcomes were assessed using the Speech Intelligibility Rating (SIR) and the Meaningful Use of Speech Scale (MUSS). The SIR measures the patient's ability to speak in real-life situations and classifies the patient's spontaneous speech into five categories, ranging from 1 (unintelligible) to 5 (intelligible to all listeners). The MUSS was used to determine the frequency of language use in the child's daily behavior and consisted of ten questions, scored out of 40 based on the frequency of behavior.

Closed or open-set tests were also included in some of the studies. In the closed test, the child is required to point out one of the given pictures and objects on demand. The commonly used closed-set speech perception tests are Word Intelligibility by Picture Identification, Pediatric Speech Intelligibility, etc. Open-set tests require children to repeat words or sentences. Commonly used open-set tests include the Consonant-Nucleus-Consonant (CNC) test, the multisyllabic word neighborhood test, phonological based kindergarten, etc.

8.1.2 Level of CI Outcomes

Patients with CND could benefit from CI, but outcomes were poor. Only some patients with CND could achieve open speech ability after CI, and approximately half could only achieve responsiveness to sound after CI. Young et al. classified the postoperative outcomes of patients with CND into four levels based on appropriate assessment of age and skill level, including postoperative detection thresholds, questionnaire assessment, closed- and open-set tests: level 1, non-stimulation or minimal detection; level 2, improved detection with apparent perceiving benefit; level 3, closed-set speech perception; or level 4, open-set speech perception (Young et al. 2012). They found that of the 10 patients with CND in the study, three patients belonged to level 1, three to level 2, one to level 3, and three to level 4.

In 2017, Peng et al. summarized 18 studies that described CI outcomes of 91 patients with CND (Peng et al. 2017). They reported that almost all studies had patients with CND who achieved level 3 or 4. In 10 of the 18 studies, at least one patient achieved open-set speech perception. Overall, of the 91 patients, 22% (20/91) were unresponsive to sound, 32% (29/91) had improved detection, 16% (15/91) achieved closed-set speech perception, and 30% (27/91) achieved open-set speech perception.

Vesseur et al. summarized 15 studies from 2003 to 2016 with 108 patients with CND (Vesseur et al. 2018). CI outcomes in patients with CND were widely varied. Of the 108 patients with CND, 44 (41%) patients achieved only voice detection, 37 (34%) achieved closed-set speech perception, and 27 (25%) achieved open-set speech perception.

8.1.3 Comparison with Normal CN

Some studies have reported differences in CI outcomes between patients with CND and normal CN. Patients with CND had significantly poorer CI outcomes than patients with normal CN. In 2010, Woo et al. reported the CI outcomes in six children with CND (study group) and 15 patients with normal CN (control group) (Kang et al. 2010). The IT-MAIS scores of the study group did not reach the level of the control group at each follow-up time point, except for patient 6. However, most patients showed a consistent improvement, with the patient 6 score exceeding the mean of the control group. CAP scores showed a similar improvement to IT-MAIS scores, in which the study group scored higher, showing a consistent improvement, but scored lower than the control group. Patient 3 scored poorly; the score of patient 6 exceeded the mean of the control group but progressed slowly after 12 months after surgery. Three patients in the study group had an SIR score of 0 at the recent follow-up. In contrast, patients 2, 5, and 6 showed a delayed improvement. In the open-set monosyllabic word recognition test, the mean score in the control group gradually increased over time, reaching a score of ≥80% 12 months after CI. In the study group, five patients did not show detection at the last follow-up visit and six began showing delayed improvement after 18 months. The results were similar for open-set word recognition. The control group showed a consistent improvement, achieving scores >90% at 18 months. On the contrary, five patients in the study group did not show detection at the last follow-up, while six patients began to show delayed improvement after 12 months.

In 2012, Jerome et al. reported differences in Pediatric Ranked Order Speech Perception (PROSPER) scores after CI in patients with cochlear nerve hypoplasia (CNH) (study group) and patients with normal CN (control group) (Valero et al. 2012). The tests are ranked according to their relative difficulty and quantified from 0 (least complex) to 34 (most complex), allowing comparison of auditory and speech outcomes under different test conditions. The results showed that the CNH group had significantly lower PROSPER scores than the normal CN group, both at the initial test (CNH, 13.35 ± 12.25; N = 17 vs. normal CN, 21.76 ± 11.17; N = 21) and at their recent test (CNH, 18.53 ± 13.37; N = 15 vs. normal CN, 28.37 ± 11.40; N = 19). Furthermore, the study explored the relationship between PROSPER scores and CI experience. The results showed that PROSPER scores were higher in the normal CN group at all time periods than in the CNH group. Furthermore, PROSPER scores in the control group continued to improve 24 months after CI, while scores in the study group appeared to plateau after this period. Eight of the 10 children in the control group (80%) achieved a maximum score of 34. After 120 months of CI, PROSPER scores were significantly higher in the control group than in the study group. Figure 8.1 shows the mean PROSPER scores for the control and study groups with respect to the CI experience.

Medhat et al. compared CI outcomes in patients with cochlear nerve aplasia (CNA), CNH, and normal CN in 2021 (Yousef et al. 2021). Five patients with CNA, two with CNH, and 10 with normal CN were included in the study. Statistical analysis showed significant differences in MAIS scores between the three groups, with a

Fig. 8.1 Mean PROSPER scores of cochlear implantation (CI) experience for the study and control groups (reproduced with permission from Valero et al. 2012)

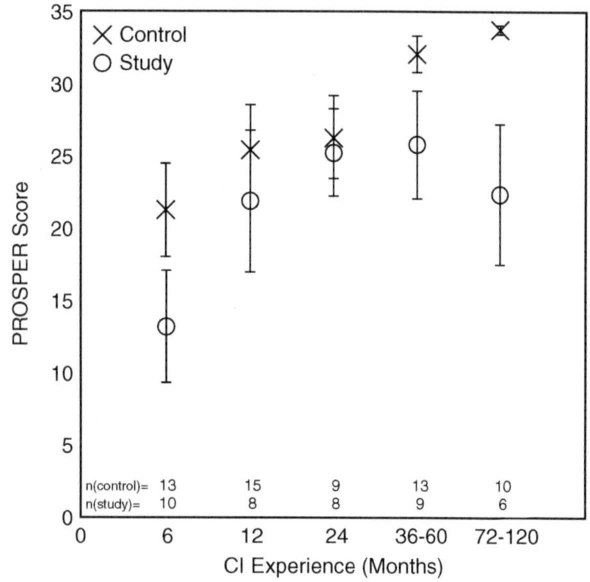

mean score of 12.50, 6.50, and 3 in the control, CNH, and CNA groups, respectively. The three groups also differed significantly in the MUSS scores, with a mean score of 11.85, 9.75, and 3 in the control, CNH, and CNA groups, respectively. Post hoc analysis showed that the control group achieved significantly better scores than the CNA group, but was comparable to the CNH group. There was no significant difference between the CNA and CNH groups. The mean speech awareness threshold (SAT) of the children in the three groups showed a significant difference, and the SAT of the control group was significantly lower than that of the CNH and CNA groups; however, no differences in threshold were found between the two groups (CAN and CNH).

8.2 Radiological Factor

Radiology plays an important role in diagnosis due to its non-invasiveness and simplicity. The diagnosis of CND is mainly based on 3D-MRI. Measurement of the CN area on MRI is the most direct way to determine the CN status. However, the CN is difficult to see due to the limited resolution of the current MRI. Sennaroglu et al. (Freeman and Sennaroglu 2018) summarized four reasons the CN is not visible on MRI. First, artifacts may interfere with the visualization of CN due to patient movement. Second, the nearby vessels and cerebellum may obscure the nerve. Third, it is difficult to visualize the CNs, as CND is often associated with temporal bone abnormalities, such as the narrow internal auditory canal (IAC) or bony cochlear nerve canal (BCNC). Finally, in some cases, the CN may be deformed against the wall of the IAC or may not be separated from the VCN or travel outside the IAC. Due to the limited ability of MRI to identify the CN, CN fibers may still be present when the CN nerve is not visible on MRI. Therefore, multiple radiological factors are considered in decision-making. This part focuses on the role of radiological factors in the diagnosis of CND and summarizes their relationship with CI outcomes in patients with CND.

8.2.1 IAC

The diameter of the IAC is measured in the axial position with high-resolution computed tomography, with the maximum diameter measured at the midpoint of the IAC (Fig. 8.2). The diameter of the IAC midpoint indirectly reflects the number of CN fibers.

IAC stenosis is generally defined as the diameter of the IAC midpoint <2 mm (Sennaroglu 2010). IAC stenosis is generally considered associated with CNH or CNA; Jackler et al. suggested that stenotic IAC (<1.5 mm) should be a contraindication to CI (Jackler et al. 1987). Shelton et al. first suggested that poor CI outcomes in patients with stenotic IAC (1–2 mm) were due to CND (Shelton et al. 1989). Ninety-two percent of IAC malformations are associated with VCN deficiency, and only 8% had visible VCN and facial nerve (FN) at the cerebellopontine angle (CPA) (Giesemann et al. 2012). However, several recent studies have shown that a narrow IAC is not always indicative of CND. Adunka et al. reported that 56% of patients with CNA had normal IAC (Adunka et al. 2006); Yan et al. reported that 53% of patients with CND had normal IAC (diameter >3 mm) (Yan et al. 2013). These results suggest that IAC stenosis is a poor indicator of CND.

The stenotic IAC suggests that the prediction of postoperative CI outcomes is possible, but the correlation is not clear, which is consistent with the CN condition. Kari et al. found that the diameter of the IAC midpoint is a predictor of positive hearing outcomes (Kari et al. 2022). However, Han et al. measured the diameter of the IAC in 25 patients with CND and found that the diameter of the IAC midpoint did not correlate significantly with the CAP and IT-MAIS scores 2 years after CI (Han et al. 2019). The effectiveness of the diameter of the IAC midpoint as a single radiological factor in predicting CI outcomes is limited.

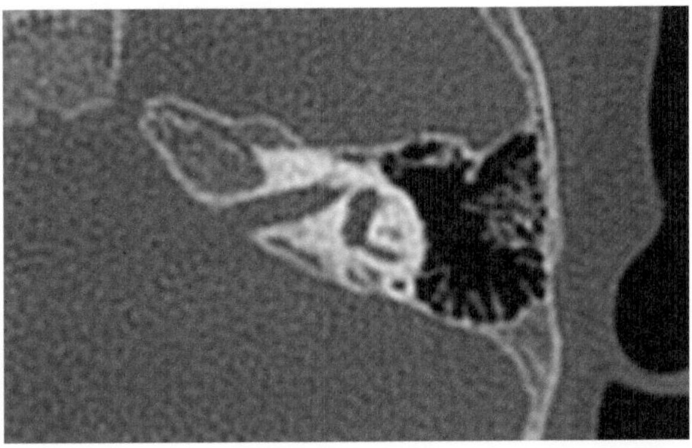

Fig. 8.2 Measurement of internal auditory canal diameter using high-resolution computed tomography (distance between the two black arrows) (reproduced with permission from Lu et al. 2022)

8.2.2 BCNC

BCNC is located between the base of the IAC and the base of the modiolus and contains CN fibers that originate from the spiral ganglion (SGN) through the IAC (Fig. 8.3). The BCNC diameter is the internal diameter of the bone wall at the base of the modiolus measured on CT. Henderson et al. evaluated histopathological sections from normal patients and the mean maximum BCNC diameter was 2.26 ± 0.25 mm (Henderson et al. 2011). Meanwhile, the BCNC diameter measured by Jang et al. in normal patients was 2.38 ± 0.28 mm (Jang et al. 2012).

Compared to IAC stenosis, BCNC stenosis is a more sensitive indicator of CND. Chung et al. found that the incidence of CND was much higher in patients with BCNC stenosis (76%) than in those with normal BCNC (21%); and the diameter of BCNC in patients with CND (1.11 mm) was significantly smaller than those with normal CN (2.08 mm) (Chung et al. 2018). However, there are no uniform criteria for BCNC stenosis. Stjernholm et al. suggested that CND should be considered when BCNC diameter <1.4 mm, which predicted poor CI outcomes (Stjernholm 2003). Komatsubara et al. suggested that CND could be observed on MRI when BCNC diameter <1.5 mm on CT (Komatsubara et al. 2007). Miyasaka et al. suggested that CNA or CNH should be considered when BCNC diameter <1.5 mm; when BCNC diameter >1.5 mm, CNH was less likely to occur (Miyasaka et al. 2010). Tahir et al. reported that only 10% of patients with BCNC <1.5 mm had normal CN (Tahir et al. 2017). Kono et al. found that BCNC diameter <1.7 mm might indicate CND (Kono 2008). Therefore, multiple values, such as 1.4 mm, 1.5 mm, and 1.7 mm, should be combined to determine BCNC stenosis to avoid omission.

The diameter of BCNC was significantly correlated with the CI outcomes. Chung et al. divided patients into three groups according to BCNC diameter: group 1, <1.4 mm; group 2, 1.4–2.0 mm; and group 3, 2.0 mm (Chung et al. 2018). The results showed that the CAP scores at 36 months after CI were significantly lower in groups 1 and 2 than in group 3, with 5.1, 5.0, and 6.4, respectively. Similarly, groups 1 and 2 performed poorly on the open-set score and picture vocabulary test.

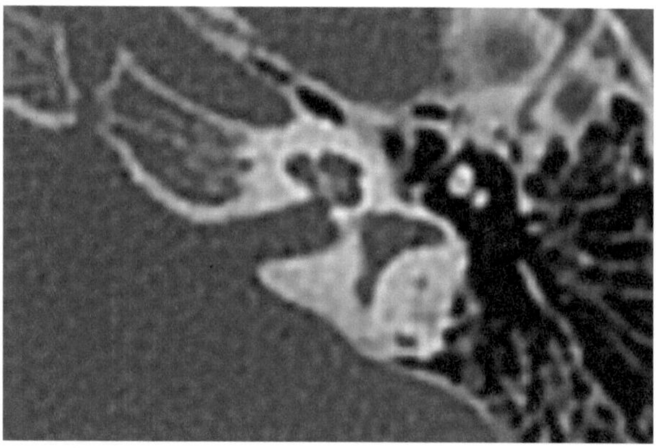

Fig. 8.3 Measurement of the bony cochlear nerve canal diameter using high-resolution computed tomography (distance between the two black arrows)

When CN was present, BCNC stenosis was not significantly correlated with CAP scores 2 years after CI, but it was positively correlated with the open-set score. Compared with IAC, BCNC has greater specificity in predicting CN and better predicting CI outcomes. Clemmens et al. reported that BCNC has a sensitivity of 84% and a specificity of 98% in its ability to diagnose CND, while IAC predicts a specificity of 98% and a sensitivity of only 44% (Clemmens et al. 2013). Therefore, the BCNC diameter can be used as a predictor of CI outcomes.

8.2.3 Vestibulocochlear Nerve and FN

The normal VCN is located posterior to the FN, and both nerves cross the CPA in a lateral-anterior direction to enter the IAC at the internal auditory meatus. Approximately 90% of the VCN separates in the middle of the IAC (Freeman and Sennaroglu 2018), forming the CN and vestibular nerve, which continue to divide into the superior vestibular nerve and inferior vestibular nerve. The VCN contains all CN fibers; therefore, it has been suggested that CND is identical to VCN deficiency or defined as the absence of VCN or thin VCN (Yamazaki et al. 2015). The VCN area can indirectly reflect the number of CNs. Thai-Van H et al. reported a patient with only FN was found on preoperative MRI, but the patient's functional MRI suggested auditory cortex activation (Van et al. 2000). Song et al. reported two patients in whom CNH was found on ABI, but VCN was not observed on preoperative MRI (Song et al. 2011). This suggests that CN fibers may still be present when CN is not visible on MRI. CI outcomes depend on the number of SGN that are available to receive electrical stimulation. Birman et al. (2016) and Kari et al. (2022) found that patients without visible CN on MRI could benefit from CI. Therefore, the invisibility of the CN on MRI may be due to the limitations of the technique.

Direct measurement of the VCN area is difficult, and some studies have chosen to measure the area ratio of VCN and FN. The VCN diameter is generally 1.5–2 times the diameter of FN, and the CN diameter is similar to FN (Fig. 8.4) (Casselman et al. 1997). Casselman et al. concluded that in the normal ear, the diameter of the VCN trunk at the CPA would not be smaller than the adjacent FN; CND was diagnosed only when the diameter of the CN was much smaller than that of the FN

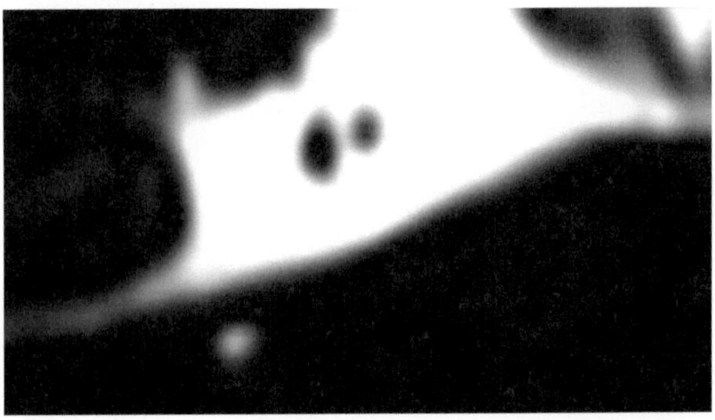

Fig. 8.4 Measurement of the area ratio of the vestibulocochlear nerve to the facial nerve at the cerebellopontine angle using magnetic resonance imaging (black arrows)

within IAC (Casselman et al. 1997). Kutz et al. defined CND as the CN diameter at the midpoint of IAC that was smaller than the adjacent FN diameter (Kutz Jr et al. 2011). Levi et al. defined it as a CN <50% of the adjacent FN (Levi et al. 2013). Casselman et al. defined CND likely to be diagnosed when CN/FN was 0.915 (Clemmens et al. 2013). Currently, the criterion to determine CND by VCN/FN or CN/FN remains unclear.

The VCN is generally larger than the FN; when the FN is larger than the VCN, the specificity of the diagnosis of CND is higher and suggests poorer CI outcomes. Yamazaki et al. reported the relationship between VCN/FN and postoperative CI outcomes; 83% of patients with IAC stenosis had FN larger than VCN; the mean postoperative CAP score in patients with FN larger than the VCN was 1.1, while the mean postoperative CAP score for CI in patients with FN smaller than the VCN was 4.1 (Yamazaki et al. 2015). Han et al. measured VCN/FN in CPA and found that VCN/FN was significantly correlated with CAP and IT-MAIS scores 2 years after CI (Han et al. 2019). The evaluation of VCN/FN was effective in predicting CI outcomes.

8.2.4 CN Classification

Because it is difficult to distinguish CN from other nerves on MRI, Birman et al. updated the CN classification based on the IAC nerve grading system (Birman et al. 2016). CNA was defined as 0, 1, 2, or 3 nerve bundles in IAC (IAC nerve class 0-III); CNH was defined as four nerve bundles, but thin CN (IAC nerve class IV); normal was defined as four nerve bundles with normal CN (IAC nerve class V) (Fig. 8.5).

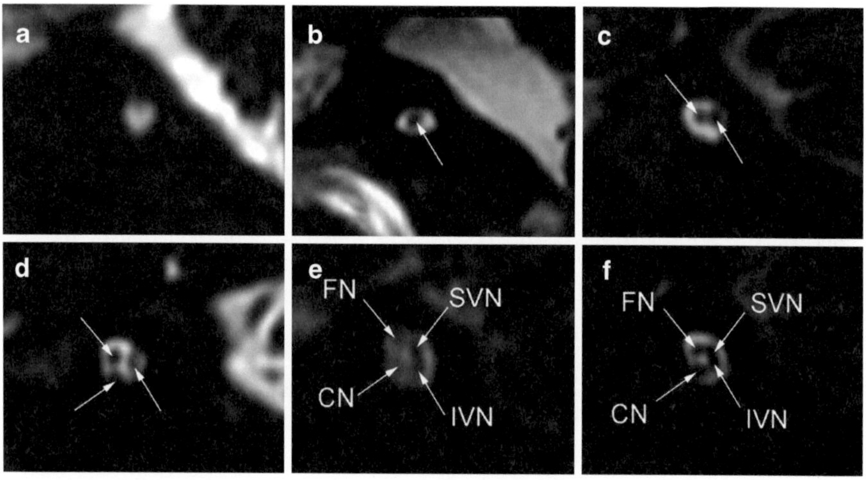

Fig. 8.5 The number of nerve bundles (indicated by white arrows) in the internal auditory canal on oblique sagittal magnetic resonance imaging. A, no nerve bundles; B, one nerve bundle; C, two nerve bundles; D, three nerve bundles; E, four nerve bundles (thin CN); F, four nerve bundles (normal CN). *CN* cochlear nerve, *FN* facial nerve, *IVN* inferior vestibular nerve, *SVN* superior vestibular nerve (reproduced with permission from Lu et al. 2022)

Under this classification system, Birman et al. reported that 47% of patients with CNA, 89% of patients with CNH, and 71% of patients with normal CN had a CAP score of 5–7 after CI. This classification was significantly and positively associated with the proportion of patients with CAP scores of 5–7 (Birman et al. 2016). Meanwhile, among patients who used spoken language as their primary mode of communication after CI, the ratio of CNH to CNA cases was 6.4, and the ratio of normal CN to CNA cases was 11, indicating a significant relationship between this classification and the primary mode of communication. Han et al. reported 25 cases and found that this classification system was significantly associated with CAP scores after CI, nine of which were grade IV. They also reported that 57.1% of grade III, 40% of grade II, 75% of grade I, and 11.1% of grade IV had CAP scores <2 at 2 years after CI (Han et al. 2019). Kari et al. reported that 63.3% of patients who did not respond to sound after CI were grade 0, and the number of nerve bundles in the IAC was associated with better hearing outcomes (Kari et al. 2022). Therefore, CN classification can effectively predict CI outcomes.

8.3 Electrophysiological Factor

CN may not show well on MRI, so the function of CN could be assessed with electrophysiological tests. Previous studies have focused on electrically evoked auditory brainstem response (EABR) and electrically evoked auditory nerve compound action potentials (ECAP).

8.3.1 EABR

EABR is an objective electrophysiological test that reflects the functional status of CN and brainstem auditory conduction pathways. Previous studies suggest that EABR was correlated with CI outcomes. Yamazaki et al. evaluated the correlation between preoperative MRI, intraoperative EABR, and 2-year postoperative CAP scores in 19 children with CND (Minami et al. 2015). All children with "CN7 > CN8/negative evoked wave V (eV)" were found to have CAP scores ≤3, while all children with "CN7 ≤ CN8/positive eV" had CAP scores ≥3. The presence of eV with typical latency suggested better CI outcomes. Wang et al. compared the EABR characteristics of 54 patients with CND and 20 patients with normal CN and analyzed the relationship between EABR and CI outcomes (Wang et al. 2022). The results showed that the detection rate of preoperative EABR in patients with normal CN was 100% and showed well-differentiated waveforms; patients with CND elicited EABR waveforms with different degrees of differentiation, and the detection rate was 88.89%. The EABR waveforms in the CND group differed significantly from those in the control group in terms of average wave V threshold, average dynamic range, and V-wave I/O curve slope. The EABR thresholds were significantly and positively correlated with the C value, wave V I/O slope, and postoperative category of auditory perception.

8.3.2 ECAP

ECAP is a near-field neural response generated by the synchronized response of CN fibers to electrical stimulation. ECAP allows a direct assessment of the neural response of the CN and better reflects the functional state of the nerve. Compared to children with normal CN, children with CND had significantly higher ECAP thresholds, smaller maximum ECAP amplitude, flatter slope of I/O function, and longer absolute refractory period (He et al. 2018). He et al. developed a prediction model for the CN index based on ECAP parameters (Skidmore et al. 2020). ECAP parameters included the refractory recovery function, ECAP threshold, the slope of I/O function, and negative-peak latency. The CN index was significantly and positively correlated with the scores of the CNC test and AzBio sentences in quiet.

8.4 CI Outcomes of CND Patients in Our Research

8.4.1 Auditory and Speech Outcomes

8.4.1.1 CND Patients

In 2017, our center reported the follow-up results of the auditory and speech outcomes of 43 patients with CND and 43 non-CND 1 year after CI (Wei et al. 2017) and reported that 35% of patients with CND combined with IEM. Auditory and speech performance was evaluated in terms of CAP, SIR, MUSS, and IT-MAIS/MAIS. This study found that patients with CND had lower mean scores on all questionnaires than non-CND patients, and there was considerable individual variation in all scores of patients with CND. The mean CAP score for patients with CND was 2.91, ranging from 0 to 7, which was significantly worse than the mean score for non-CND patients (mean, 5.98; range, 3–7). For SIR, the mean score for patients with CND (mean, 2.23; range, 1–5) was similar to non-CND patients (mean, 3.77; range, 1–5). Although IT-MAIS/MAIS scores (mean, 19.93; range, 2–39) and MUSS scores (mean, 15.23; range, 0–40) were worse in patients with CND than in non-CND patients (IT-MAIS/MAIS, mean, 28.24; range, 9–39 and MUSS, mean, 27.48; range, 1–39), there was substantial overlap in scores. Therefore, our center found that the CI outcomes were worse in patients with CND than in those without CND (Fig. 8.6).

8.4.1.2 Patients with CND with Normal Cochlea

In the aforementioned study, 35% of patients with CND combined with IEM, which may increase individual heterogeneity. Therefore, in a follow-up study, we followed the postoperative CI outcomes of patients with CND and summarized the auditory and speech performance of 70 patients with CND with normal cochlea at 2 years postoperatively. Auditory and speech performance was also evaluated in terms of CAP, SIR, IT-MAIS/MAIS, and MUSS. Patients with CND with normal cochlea had a mean CAP score of 4.10 (range, 2–7) and a mean IT-MAIS/MAIS score of

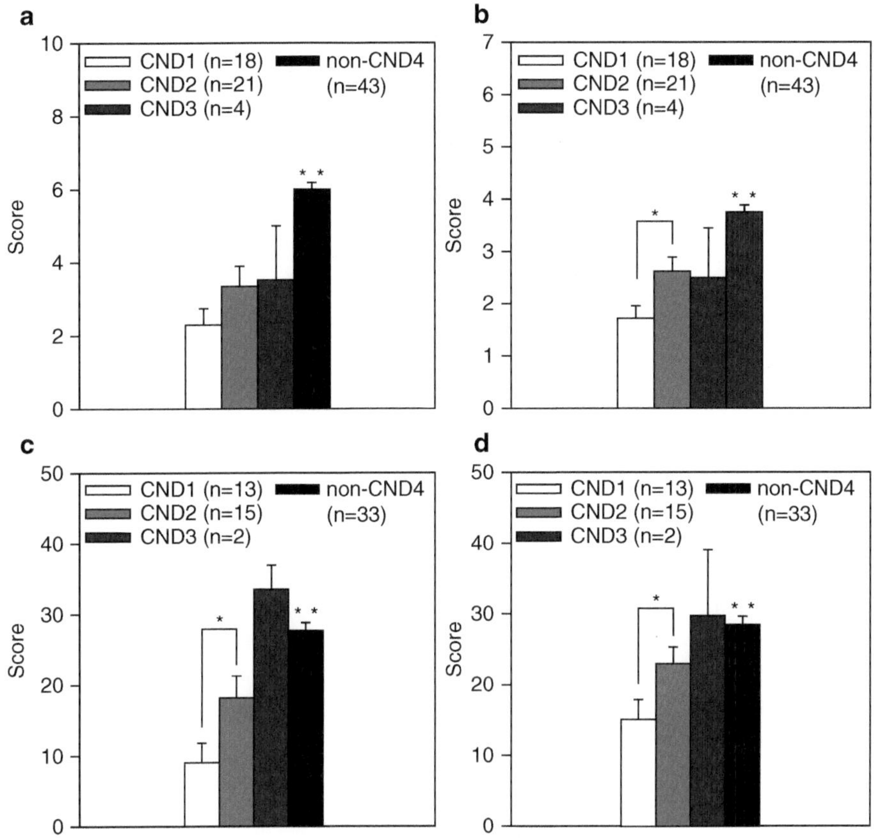

Fig. 8.6 Scores for patients with CND with one, two, or three nerve bundles (CND1, CND2, CND3, respectively) and non-CND patients with four nerve bundles (non-CND4) (reproduced with permission from Wei et al. 2017). (**a**) CAP score, (**b**) SIR score, (**c**) MUSS score, (**d**) MAIS-IT/MAIS score

25.14 (range, 3–40). For SIR and MUSS, which assess speech ability, greater variability was observed between patients, resulting in lower mean scores. The mean score for SIR was 1.87, ranging from 1 to 4, while the mean score for MUSS was 11.96, ranging from 0 to 33. Table 8.1 shows the distribution of CAP, SIR, IT-MAIS/MAIS, and MUSS.

CAP and SIR were divided into two groups respectively to differentiate auditory and speech performance. CAP were divided into understanding of some verbal language (CAP of 5–7) and no understanding of some verbal language (CAP of 0–4). SIR were divided into developing or developed intelligible speech (SIR of 2–5) and unintelligible connected speech (SIR of 1). Figure 8.7a, b show the distribution of CAP and SIR, and Fig. 8.7c, d show the grouping of CAP and SIR. Only 51.4% (36/70) of patients with CND developed spoken language understanding 2 years after CI, and only 55.7% (39/70) developed intelligible speech 2 years after CI.

Table 8.1 Descriptive statistics of patients (reproduced with permission from Lu et al. 2022)

	Count	Mean	Standard deviation	Min.	25%	50%	75%	Max.
CAP	70.00	4.10	1.32	2.00	3.00	5.00	5.00	7.00
SIR	70.00	1.87	0.92	1.00	1.00	2.00	3.00	4.00
IT-MAIS/MAIS	70.00	25.14	10.47	3.00	18.00	26.50	33.75	40.00
MUSS	70.00	11.96	10.32	0.00	3.00	8.00	21.75	33.00

8.4.1.3 CND Patients with IEM

In addition to the status of the CN, the cochlear structure also influences postoperative CI outcomes. Minami et al. (2020) classified the cochlea into four categories according to the condition of the cochlear nerve and modiolus and found that patients with grade I (modiolus present + normal CN) had significantly higher CAP scores than patients with grade II (modiolus deficiency + normal CN), grade III (modiolus present + CND), and grade IV (modiolus deficiency + CND). For patients with CND with modiolus deficiency, only 25% of the patients had a CAP score of ≥4, indicating a poorer postoperative outcome after CI. For long-term follow-up of CI outcomes in patients with CND with severe IEM, we followed up on 67 patients using questionnaires.

According to Sennaroglu's 2017 classification of IEM (Aldhafeeri and Alsanosi 2017), complete labyrinthine aplasia, rudimentary otocyst, and cochlear aplasia are definite indications of auditory brainstem implant (ABI). CI is preferred for common cavity (CC), cochlear hypoplasia (CH), incomplete partition type I (IP-I), and CND. The side with better CN development or better residual hearing was chosen as the CI ear; if the patient could not benefit from CI, ABI was performed contralaterally. Modiolus deficiency malformations suitable for CI include CC, CH (CH-I and CH-II), and IP-I (Fig. 8.8).

A total of 60 patients were included in this study; 31 (51.67%) were male and 29 (49.33%) were female. Each group had 20 patients. Questionnaires were used to evaluate auditory and speech CI outcomes at onset and 12, 24, and 36 months after onset. Auditory outcomes were assessed using CAP and IT-MAIS/MAIS scores. Speech effects were assessed using the SIR and MUSS scores. Simultaneously, closed bisyllabic speech tests were performed in a quiet environment for some children who were able and cooperative.

A total of 60 patients participated in the assessment at onset and 12 months after onset, 58 patients at 24 months, and 51 patients at 36 months. Overall, 80.4% (41/51) of the patients were able to understand some spoken language (CAP >4) and 68.6% (35/51) developed an intelligible language (SIR >1) at 36 months after switch-on. The scores for each type at each time period are shown in Fig. 8.9.

During follow-up, some children completed the closed-set test in a quiet environment and cooperated with the test. The median closed speech recognition rate was 50% for patients with CH and 23.3% for CC (Table 8.2).

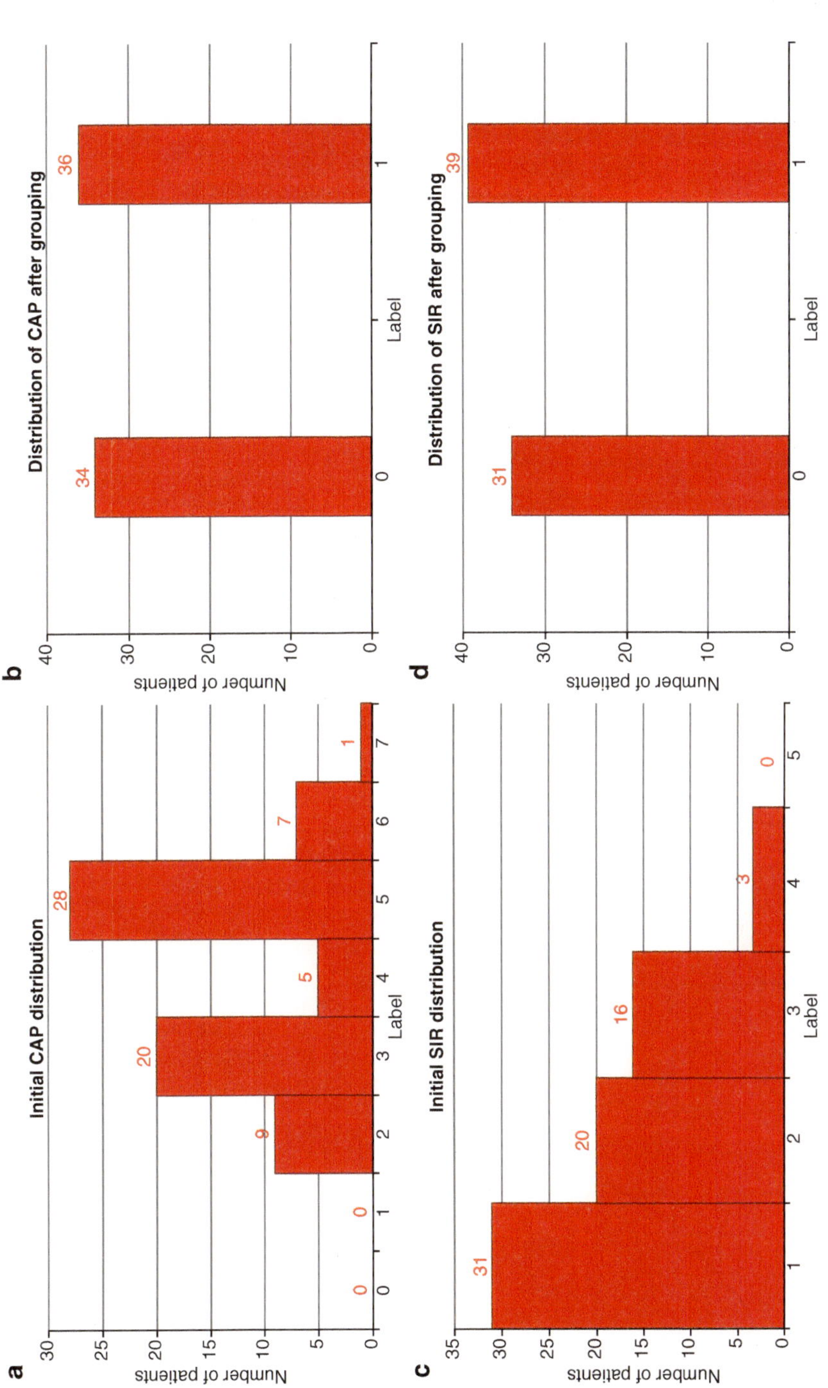

Fig. 8.7 Patient distribution before and after considering the CAP and SIR grouping (reproduced with permission from Lu et al. 2022)

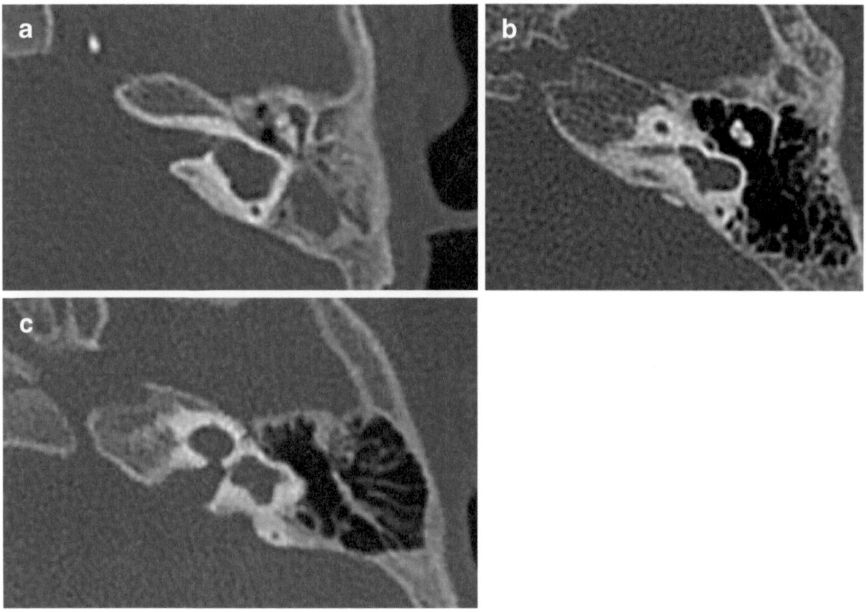

Fig. 8.8 (**a**) Common cavity. (**b**) Cochlear hypoplasia. (**c**) Incomplete partition-I

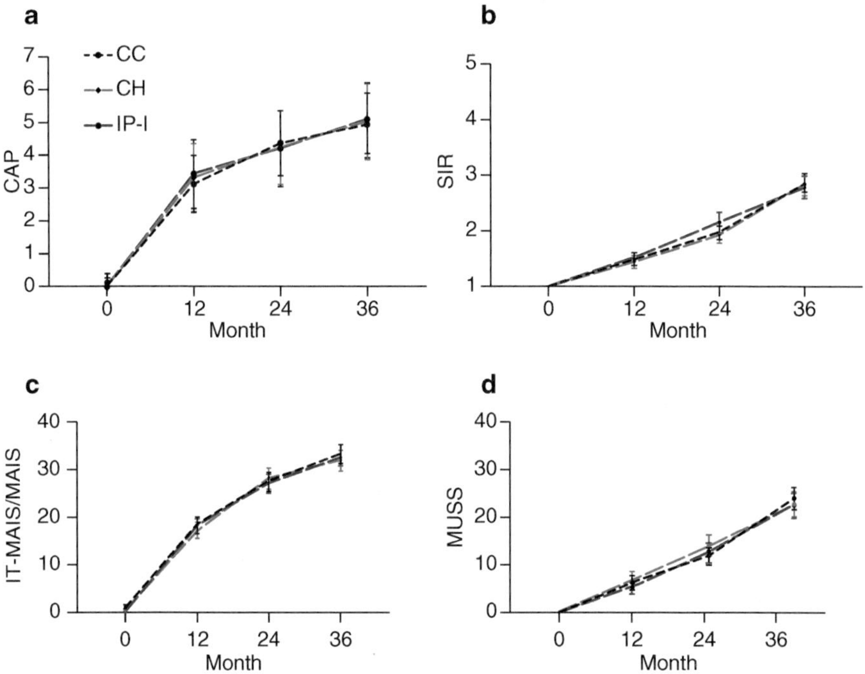

Fig. 8.9 (**a**) Development of CAP scores in different groups by modiolar deficiency-type malformation. *CC* common cavity, *CH* cochlear hypoplasia, *IP-I* incomplete partition-I (IP); Normal, normal cochlea. (**b**) Development of SIR scores. (**c**) Development of IT-MAIS/MAIS scores. (**d**) Development of MUSS scores

Table 8.2 Closed-set recognition rate

Number	Cochlea	Closed-set recognition rate	Median
1	IP-I	100%	/
2	CH	100%	50%
3	CH	80%	
4	CH	50%	
5	CH	40%	
6	CH	26.70%	
7	CC	63.30%	23.3%
8	CC	33.30%	
9	CC	13.30%	
10	CC	6.60%	

8.4.2 Preoperative Factors Associated with Auditory and Speech Outcomes

8.4.2.1 CND Patients

In our 2017 study, we explored preoperative radiological indicators that predicted postoperative outcomes after CI in patients with CND (Wei et al. 2017). IAC diameter, BCNC diameter, and the number of nerve bundles were included in multiple linear regression. The results showed that IAC diameter had no effect on the CAP, SIR, IT-MAIS/MAIS, and MUSS scores in patients with CND after surgery. BCNC diameter was significantly and positively correlated with the SIR and IT-MAIS/MAIS scores in patients with CND. Similarly, the number of nerve bundles was significantly and positively correlated with the MUSS scores. When both BCNC diameter and the number of nerve bundles were considered, the predictive effect of these two indicators on IT-MAIS/MAIS and MUSS scores was greatly improved in patients with CND. This suggests that the combination of BCNC diameter and the number of nerve bundles effectively predicts auditory and speech outcomes in patients with CND after CI.

8.4.2.2 CND Patients with Normal Cochlea

In the follow-up study, the number of patients increased, along with large individual differences; therefore, we used machine learning to develop a predictive model for the auditory and speech outcomes of patients with CND 2 years after CI. Auditory performance was assessed using the CAP score, which classified the patients into spoken language understanding (CAP of 5–7) and no spoken language understanding (CAP of 0–4). Speech ability was assessed using the SIR score and the patients were classified as having intelligible speech (SIR of 2–5) and unintelligible speech (SIR of 1). CI outcomes depend on many factors, which are very complex. Taking into account the experience of previous studies, we collected information on the age at implantation, radiological characteristics, and audiological characteristics of patients with CND. Radiological characteristics include BCNC diameter, IAC diameter, number of nerve bundles, area ratio of the VCN to the FN, and VCN area. Audiological characteristics included mean residual

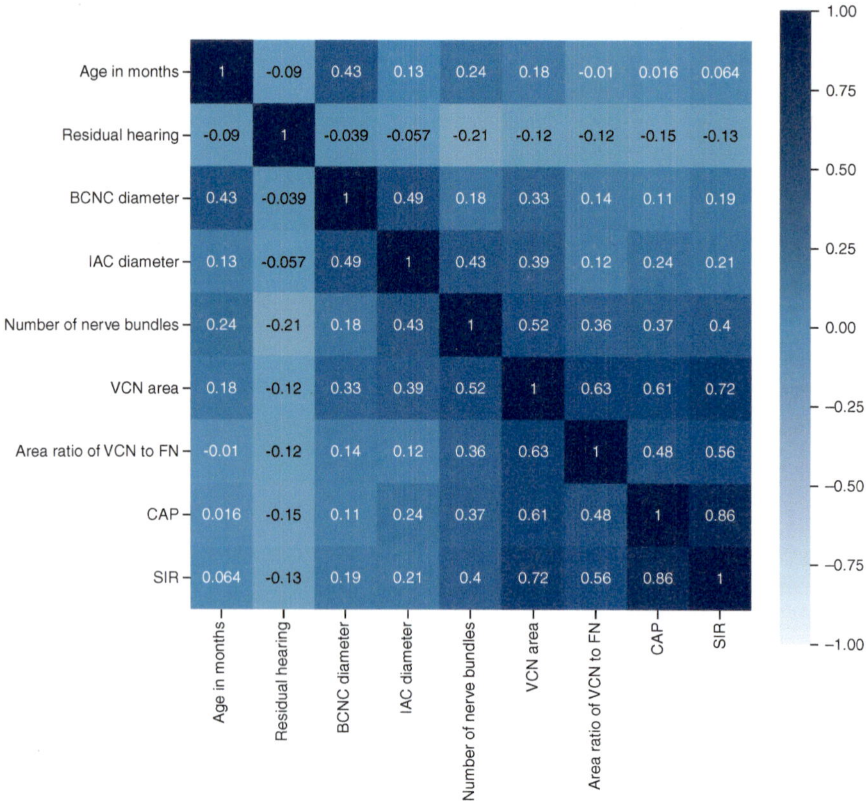

Fig. 8.10 Correlation coefficient matrix (reproduced with permission from Lu et al. 2022)

hearing threshold, 40 Hz, ABR, CM, DPOAE, and acoustic conduction resistance. The correlation coefficient matrix is shown in Fig. 8.10. Considering the high correlation coefficient between the area ratio of VCN to FN and VCN area (0.63), the area ratio of VCN to FN is removed. Data-driven methods, including stability selection and parameter-optimized support vector machine (SVM), were applied to the data of patients with CND to investigate the effect of various factors on CI outcomes and to build a predictive model.

Stability selection is a machine learning method that identifies highly consistent data features and is used to examine which factors best distinguish the postoperative hearing speech outcomes of patients with CND after CI, helping to select the most important and consistent features. We measured and averaged the audiological and radiological features of the patients to form feature vectors. The feature scores were scaled between 0 and 1, where 0 was the lowest score (irrelevant feature) and 1 was the highest score (most representative or stable feature). Stability selection provided the overall feature scores (0–1) based on the selected frequency and was used to select the most important and consistent features over a range of model parameters.

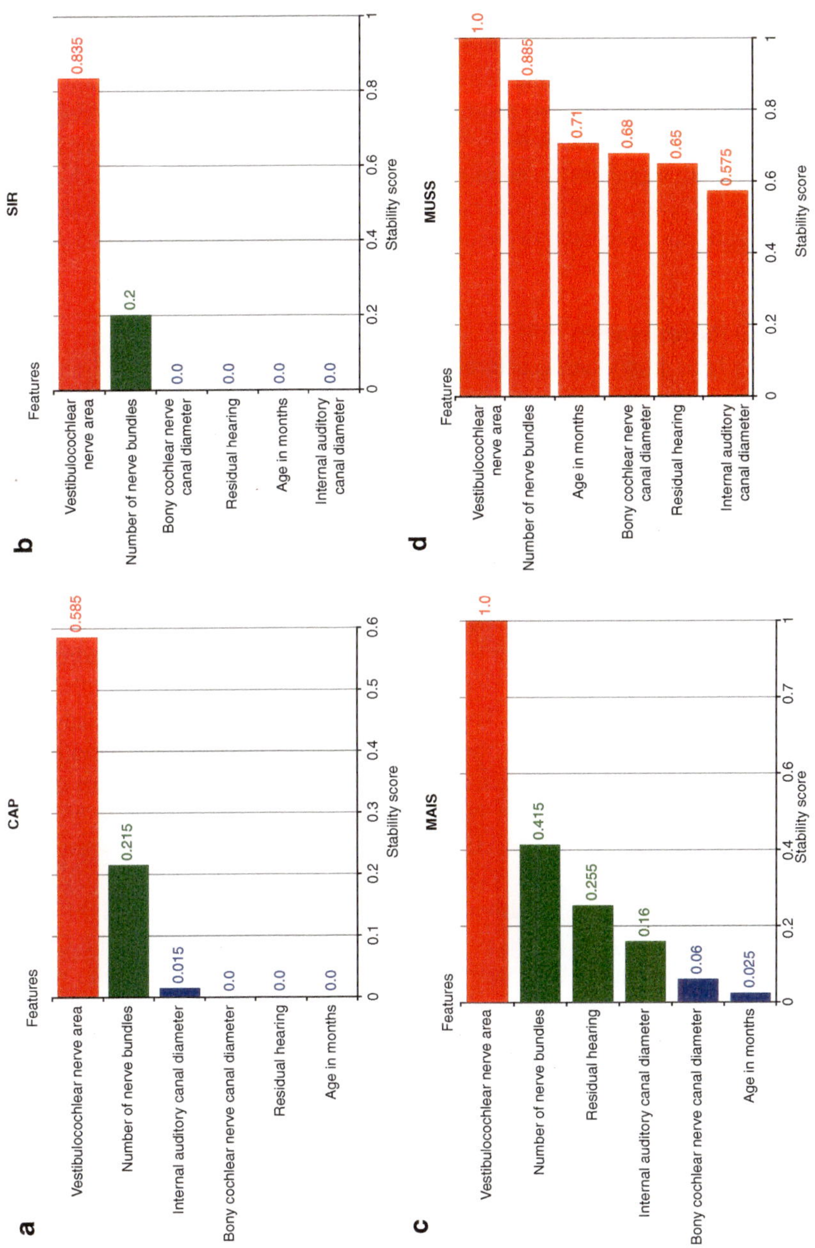

Fig. 8.11 Stability scores for feature selection (reproduced with permission from Lu et al. 2022). Effect of features on **(a)** SIR, **(b)** CAP, **(c)** IT-MAIS/MAIS, and **(d)** MUSS

As shown in Fig. 8.11, for CAP, stability was obtained in descending order for the VCN area, number of nerve bundles, IAC diameter, BCNC diameter, residual hearing, and age at implantation; for SIR, this order was obtained for the VCN area, number of nerve bundles, BCNC diameter, residual hearing, the age at implantation, and IAC diameter. We also analyzed the IT-MAIS/MAIS and MUSS scores. For the IT-MAIS/MAIS score, it was found that the VCN area was the most stable, followed by the number of nerve bundles, residual hearing, and diameter of IAC. For the MUSS score, the VCN area was the most stable factor with a stability score of 1, followed by the number of nerve bundles. Therefore, we conclude that the characteristics of the VCN area and the number of nerve bundles are the most stable and have the greatest impact on auditory speech outcomes in patients with CND 2 years after CI.

8.4.2.3 CND Patients with IEM

The modiolus is an important structure in the cochlea, and when the modiolus is deficient, the cochlear structure often presents as a sac-like shape that affects the placement of electrodes. Therefore, in patients with CND with modiolus deficiency, it is unclear whether the type of cochlea or the degree of neurodevelopment affects CI outcomes.

Our research included 60 patients with modiolus deficiency, grouped according to cochlear type and neurodevelopmental degree. In a previous study of patients with CND with normal cochlea, we have found that the number of nerve bundles and VCN areas are most associated with the CI outcomes. However, in modiolus deficiency, the nerve in the CPA is difficult to measure; therefore, only the number of nerve bundles was chosen to assess the CN status. Cochlear types were divided into three groups: CC, CH, and IP-I. The number of nerve bundles was divided into one nerve bundle, two nerve bundles, three nerve bundles, and four nerve bundles in IAC. Among the malformation groups, no significant differences were shown in all scores. The comparison of outcomes between the number of nerve bundle groups evaluated by CAP, SIR, IT-MAIS/MAIS, and MUSS scores showed significant differences in all scores at 12, 24, and 36 months after CI.

The development of postoperative CAP, SIR, IT-MAIS/MAIS, and MUSS scores for each nerve bundle group is shown in Fig. 8.12. Specifically, the CAP, SIR, IT-MAIS/MAIS, and MUSS scores of patients with one nerve bundle were significantly poorer than those of patients with two nerve bundles, three nerve bundles, and four nerve bundles at 12, 24, and 36 months after CI. The SIR and MUSS scores at 24 months after CI were significantly lower in patients with one nerve bundle, two nerve bundles, and three nerve bundles than patients with four nerve bundles.

Our study found that the number of nerve bundles was significantly correlated with auditory and speech outcomes at 12, 24, and 36 months after CI, while cochlear malformation was weakly correlated with CI outcomes.

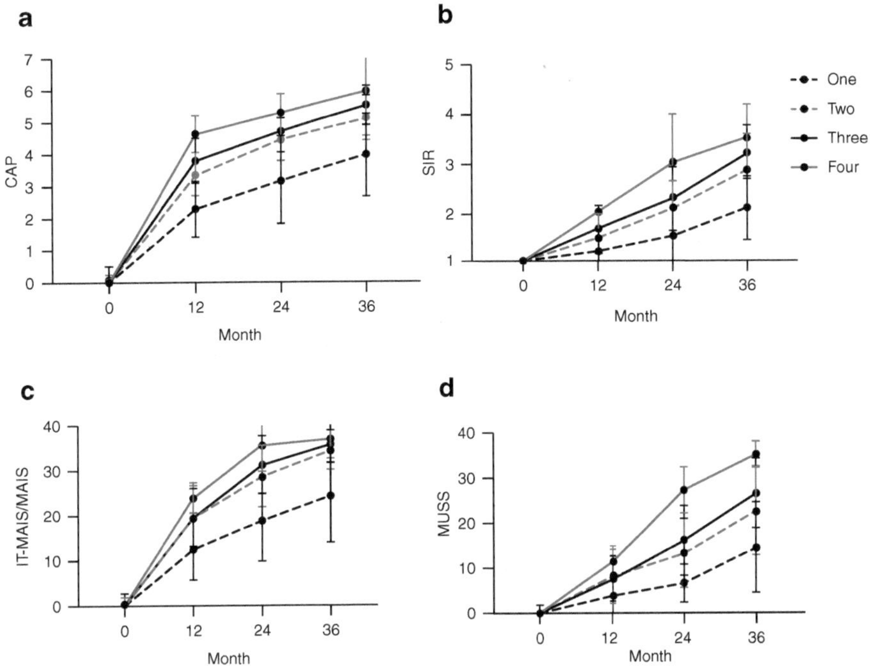

Fig. 8.12 (**a**) Development of CAP scores in different groups by the number of nerve bundles. Normal, patients without CND; (**b**) SIR score; (**c**) IT-MAIS/MAIS score; (**d**) development of the MUSS score

8.4.3 Machine Learning-Based Prediction of CI Outcomes in CND Patients with Normal Cochlea

Based on the stability selection feature, we built prediction models for CAP and SIR for patients with CND 2 years after CI using SVM. SVM classified patients with CND with characteristics of different stability thresholds and was more suitable to build classification models for small samples, which could predict CI outcomes based on preoperative data from patients with CND. The effect of the stability selection threshold on classification performance is shown in Fig. 8.13a for CAP and Fig. 8.13b for SIR. For CAP, the maximum classification performance was achieved with an accuracy of 71% at a stability score threshold of 0.10. The VCN area and the number of neural bundles were selected for this threshold. For SIR, stability selection selected two features (29%), the VCN area and the number of neural bundles, with 93% accuracy. Furthermore, even when we chose a stability threshold of 0.5 (a more conservative feature selection), only the VCN area was selected for both the CAP and SIR models. In the VCN area, the model predicts the CAP group with 64% accuracy and the SIR group with 57% accuracy. These results suggest that the use of only a few features can predict postoperative auditory and speech CI outcomes in patients with CND with a normal cochlea.

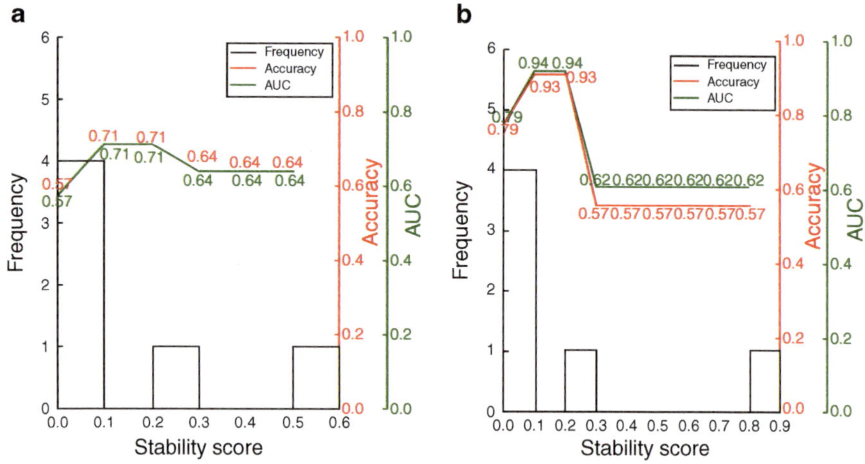

Fig. 8.13 Effect of stability score threshold on model performance for (**a**) CAP and (**b**) SIR (reproduced with permission from Lu et al. 2022). The stability score ranges from 0 to 1. AUC, area under the curve

8.5 Conclusion

CI outcomes of patients with CND vary widely, and only some patients can achieve open speech ability. CI outcomes for patients with CND are worse than those of normal CN. Radiological and electrophysiological factors were correlated with the CI outcomes of patients with CND.

References

Adunka OF, Roush PA, Teagle HFB, Brown CJ, Zdanski CJ, Jewells V, Buchman CA. Internal auditory canal morphology in children with cochlear nerve deficiency. Otology and Neurotology. 2006;27(6):793–801.

Aldhafeeri AM, Alsanosi AA. Management of surgical difficulties during cochlear implant with inner ear anomalies. Int J Pediatr Otorhinolaryngol. 2017;92:45–9.

Birman CS, Powell HRF, Gibson WPR, Elliott EJ. Cochlear implant outcomes in cochlea nerve aplasia and hypoplasia. Otol Neurotol. 2016;37(5):438–45.

Casselman JW, Offeciers FE, Govaerts PJ, Kuhweide R, Geldof H, Somers T, D'Hont G. Aplasia and hypoplasia of the vestibulocochlear nerve: diagnosis with MR imaging. Radiology. 1997;202(3):773–81.

Chung J, Jang JH, Chang SO, Song JJ, Cho SW, Kim SY, Lee JH, Oh SH. Does the width of the bony cochlear nerve canal predict the outcomes of cochlear implantation? BioMed Res Int. 2018;2018:5675848.

Clemmens CS, Guidi J, Caroff A, Cohn SJ, Brant JA, Laury AM, Bilaniuk LT, Germiller JA. Unilateral cochlear nerve deficiency in children. Otolaryngol Head Neck Surg (United States). 2013;149(2):318–25.

Freeman SR, Sennaroglu L. Management of cochlear nerve hypoplasia and aplasia. Adv Otorhinolaryngol. 2018;81:81–92.

Giesemann AM, Kontorinis G, Jan Z, Lenarz T, Lanfermann H, Goetz F. The vestibulocochlear nerve: aplasia and hypoplasia in combination with inner ear malformations. Eur Radiol. 2012;22(3):519–24.

Han JJ, Suh MW, Park MK, Koo JW, Lee JH, Oh SH. A predictive model for Cochlear implant outcome in children with Cochlear nerve deficiency. Sci Rep. 2019;9(1):1154.

He S, Shahsavarani BS, McFayden TC, Wang H, Gill KE, Xu L, Chao X, Luo J, Wang R, He N. Responsiveness of the electrically stimulated Cochlear nerve in children with Cochlear nerve deficiency. Ear Hear. 2018;39(2):238–50.

Henderson E, Wilkins A, Huang L, Kenna M, Gopen Q. Histopathologic investigation of the dimensions of the cochlear nerve canal in normal temporal bones. Int J Pediatr Otorhinolaryngol. 2011;75(4):464–7.

Jackler RK, Luxford WM, House WF. Sound detection with the cochlear implant in five ears of four children with congenital malformations of the cochlea. Laryngoscope. 1987;97(40 S):15–7.

Jang JH, Kim JH, Yoo JC, Kim CH, Kim MS, Chang SO, Oh SH, Lee JH. Implication of bony cochlear nerve canal on hearing in patients with congenital unilateral sensorineural hearing loss. Audiol Neurootol. 2012;17(5):282–9.

Kang WS, Lee JH, Lee HN, Lee KS. Cochlear implantations in young children with cochlear nerve deficiency diagnosed by MRI. Otolaryngol Head Neck Surg. 2010;143(1):101–8.

Kari E, Gillard DM, Chuang N, Go JL. Can imaging predict hearing outcomes in children with Cochleovestibular nerve abnormalities? Laryngoscope. 2022;132(Suppl 8):S1–s15.

Komatsubara S, Haruta A, Nagano Y, Kodama T. Evaluation of cochlear nerve imaging in severe congenital sensorineural hearing loss. ORL J Otorhinolaryngol Relat Spec. 2007;69(3): 198–202.

Kono T. Computed tomographic features of the bony canal of the cochlear nerve in pediatric patients with unilateral sensorineural hearing loss. Radiat Med. 2008;26(3):115–9.

Kutz JW Jr, Lee KH, Isaacson B, Booth TN, Sweeney MH, Roland PS. Cochlear implantation in children with cochlear nerve absence or deficiency. Otol Neurotol. 2011;32(6):956–61.

Levi J, Ames J, Bacik K, Drake C, Morlet T, O'Reilly RC. Clinical characteristics of children with cochlear nerve dysplasias. Laryngoscope. 2013;123(3):752–6.

Lu S, Xie J, Wei X, Kong Y, Chen B, Chen J, Zhang L, Yang M, Xue S, Shi Y, Liu S, Xu T, Dong R, Chen X, Li Y, Wang H. Machine learning-based prediction of the outcomes of cochlear implantation in patients with cochlear nerve deficiency and normal cochlea: a 2-year follow-up of 70 children. Front Neurosci. 2022;16:895560.

Minami SB, Takegoshi H, Shinjo Y, Enomoto C, Kaga K. Usefulness of measuring electrically evoked auditory brainstem responses in children with inner ear malformations during cochlear implantation. Acta Otolaryngol. 2015;135(10):1007–15.

Minami SB, Yamamoto N, Hosoya M, Enomoto C, Kaga K. Cochlear implantation in cases of inner ear malformation: a novel and simple grading, intracochlear EABR, and outcomes of hearing. Otol Neurotol. 2020;42(2):e117–23. American Neurotology Society [and] European Academy of Otology and Neurotology.

Miyasaka M, Nosaka S, Morimoto N, Taiji H, Masaki H. CT and MR imaging for pediatric cochlear implantation: emphasis on the relationship between the cochlear nerve canal and the cochlear nerve. Pediatr Radiol. 2010;40(9):1509–16.

Peng KA, Kuan EC, Hagan S, Wilkinson EP, Miller ME. Cochlear nerve aplasia and hypoplasia: predictors of Cochlear implant success. Otolaryngol Head Neck Surg. 2017;157(3):392–400.

Sennaroglu L. Cochlear implantation in inner ear malformations — a review article. Cochlear Implants Int. 2010;11(1):4–41.

Shelton C, Luxford WM, Tonokawa LL, Lo WWM, House WF. The narrow internal auditory canal in children: a contraindication to cochlear implants. Otolaryngol Head Neck Surg. 1989;100(3):227–31.

Skidmore J, Xu L, Chao X, Riggs WJ, Pellittieri A, Vaughan C, Ning X, Wang R, Luo J, He S. Prediction of the functional status of the Cochlear nerve in individual Cochlear implant users using machine learning and electrophysiological measures. Ear Hear. 2020;42(1):180–92.

Song MH, Kim SC, Kim J, Chang JW, Lee WS, Choi JY. The cochleovestibular nerve identified during auditory brainstem implantation in patients with narrow internal auditory canals: can preoperative evaluation predict cochleovestibular nerve deficiency? Laryngoscope. 2011;121(8):1773–9.

Stjernholm C. Aspects of temporal bone anatomy and pathology in conjunction with cochlear implant surgery. Acta Radiol. 2003;44(SUPPL. 430):2–15.

Tahir E, Bajin MD, Atay G, Mocan BO, Sennaroğlu L. Bony cochlear nerve canal and internal auditory canal measures predict cochlear nerve status. J Laryngol Otol. 2017;131(8):676–83.

Valero J, Blaser S, Papsin BC, James AL, Gordon KA. Electrophysiologic and behavioral outcomes of cochlear implantation in children with auditory nerve hypoplasia. Ear Hear. 2012;33(1):3–18.

Van HT, Fraysse B, Berry I, Berges C, Deguine O, Honegger A, Sevely A, Ibarrola D. Functional magnetic resonance imaging may avoid misdiagnosis of cochleovestibular nerve aplasia in congenital deafness. Am J Otol. 2000;21(5):663–70.

Vesseur A, Free R, Snels C, Dekker F, Mylanus E, Verbist B, Frijns J. Hearing restoration in Cochlear nerve deficiency: the choice between Cochlear implant or auditory brainstem implant, a meta-analysis. Otol Neurotol. 2018;39(4):428–37.

Wang B, Guo X, Cao K, Wei C, Gao Z, Wang S. Evaluation of auditory pathway by EABR before cochlear implantation and the postoperative effect analysis. Eur Arch Otorhinolaryngol. 2022; https://doi.org/10.1007/s00405-022-07458-9.

Wei X, Li Y, Chen B, Gong Y, Fu QJ, Liu T, Cui D, Su Q, Shi Y. Predicting auditory outcomes from radiological imaging in Cochlear implant patients with Cochlear nerve deficiency. Otol Neurotol. 2017;38(5):685–93.

Wu CM, Lee LA, Chen CK, Chan KC, Tsou YT, Ng SH. Impact of cochlear nerve deficiency determined using 3-dimensional magnetic resonance imaging on hearing outcome in children with cochlear implants. Otol Neurotol. 2015;36(1):14–21.

Yamazaki H, Leigh J, Briggs R, Naito Y. Usefulness of MRI and EABR testing for predicting CI outcomes immediately after Cochlear implantation in cases with Cochlear nerve deficiency. Otol Neurotol. 2015;36(6):977–84.

Yan F, Li J, Xian J, Wang Z, Mo L. The cochlear nerve canal and internal auditory canal in children with normal cochlea but cochlear nerve deficiency. Acta Radiol. 2013;54(3):292–8.

Young NM, Kim FM, Ryan ME, Tournis E, Yaras S. Pediatric cochlear implantation of children with eighth nerve deficiency. Int J Pediatr Otorhinolaryngol. 2012;76(10):1442–8.

Yousef M, Mesallam TA, Garadat SN, Almasaad A, Alzhrani F, Alsanosi A, Hagr A. Audiologic outcome of Cochlear implantation in children with Cochlear nerve deficiency. Otol Neurotol. 2021;42(1):38–46.

9 Vestibular and Balance Function of Patients with Cochlear Nerve Deficiency

Xinxing Fu, Mengya Shen, Shujin Xue, and Xingmei Wei

9.1 Vestibular Function Assessment Methods

The standard vestibular function testing battery includes caloric testing (Shepard and Jacobson 2016) and rotatory testing (Baloh et al. 1979), both focusing on the horizontal semicircular canal, and a video head impulse test (vHIT) (Halmagyi et al. 2001), which has been used to evaluate the horizontal and vertical semicircular canals. Methods to investigate the otolith organs include vestibular evoked myogenic potentials (VEMPs) (Colebatch et al. 1994; Rosengren et al. 2005) and subjective visual vertical or subjective visual horizontal (Dyde et al. 2006). This combination of tests will provide a comprehensive assessment of the complex vestibular organ. Furthermore, questionnaires, such as the dizziness handicap inventory (DHI) for adults (Jacobson and Newman 1990) and the pediatric vestibular symptom questionnaire (PVSQ) for children (Pavlou et al. 2016), were used to assess vestibular function.

X. Fu (✉)
Beijing Institute of Otolaryngology, Beijing Tongren Hospital, Capital Medical University, Beijing, China

Key Laboratory of Otolaryngology Head and Neck Surgery (Capital Medical University), Ministry of Education, Beijing, China

M. Shen · S. Xue · X. Wei
Key Laboratory of Otolaryngology Head and Neck Surgery (Capital Medical University), Ministry of Education, Beijing, China

Department of Otorhinolaryngology Head and Neck Surgery, Beijing Tongren Hospital, Capital Medical University, Beijing, China

Y. Li (ed.), *Cochlear Implantation for Cochlear Nerve Deficiency*,
https://doi.org/10.1007/978-981-19-5892-2_9

9.1.1 Caloric Test

The caloric test evaluates the responses of the horizontal semicircular canals at very low frequencies. Several studies have compared the effect of cochlear implantation (CI) surgery on vestibular function. In a meta-analysis by Ibrahim et al. (2017), a significant effect of CI surgery on the results of the caloric test was revealed; the risk ratio was 0.28. A wide variety of negative effects after CI surgery in children was reported on caloric tests (0–30%) (Jacot et al. 2009; Ajalloueyan et al. 2017).

9.1.2 Video Head Impulse Test (vHIT)

The vHIT is a quantitative test that can detect overt and covert saccades and investigate the gain in the vestibulo-ocular reflex (VOR) of each semicircular canal. A meta-analysis of five studies reported a nonsignificant effect of CI surgery on the HIT test and a low-risk ratio (0.10) (Ibrahim et al. 2017). In another meta-analysis, Abouzayd et al. determined the best testing protocol for the assessment of vestibular function after CI surgery by respectively calculating true positive, false positive, true negative, and false negative of various vestibular tests; the sensitivity of the caloric test, cVEMP, and vHIT was 21%, 32%, and 50%, respectively (Abouzayd et al. 2017).

9.1.3 Vestibular Evoked Myogenic Potential (VEMP)

Cervical VEMP (cVEMP) is based on the vestibulocollic reflex to measure the function of the saccular and inferior vestibular nerve through the ipsilateral sternocleidomastoid muscle. Ocular VEMP (oVEMP) uses vestibulo-ocular projections to assess utricular and superior vestibular nerve function by contralateral activation of the inferior oblique eye muscle. The cVEMP test was the most frequently affected by CI surgery among vestibular function tests, but the rate of negative effects varied (20–100%) (Bogle 2010; Psillas et al. 2014). The potential reason for the difference may be its anatomical proximity to the round window; therefore, the saccule may be more vulnerable to insertion injury. However, another reason is that packing during implantation may cause conductive hearing loss, which will directly impact the elicitation of VEMPs (Melvin et al. 2009).

9.1.4 Dizziness Handicap Inventory (DHI)

The DHI consists of 25 items, with the sum of the scale responses yielding a total score of (0–100 points), with higher scores indicating a more severe handicap. The scale was designed to assess three multiple sub-domains of subjective complaints about dizziness and consists of seven physical, nine functional, and nine emotional questions. Several studies have assessed vertigo and balance symptoms in patients after CI using DHI. A meta-analysis revealed a nonsignificant effect of CI surgery on DHI scores (Ibrahim et al. 2017). In most studies, the increase in DHI scores did not result in a change that required further intervention.

9.1.5 Pediatric Vestibular Symptom Questionnaire (PVSQ)

PVSQ is a scale that assesses the severity of vestibular symptoms in children aged 6–17 years. This questionnaire contains 11 questions (10 multiple-choice questions and 1 subjective question). In a study that uses PVSQ to evaluate vertigo symptoms after CI surgery, there were no significant differences in PVSQ scores between pre-implantation and post-implantation for unilateral CI in children. Only PVSQ scores in children with bilateral CI increased on day 3 post-CI but decreased on day 30, which implied that the alterations could be a transient reaction to trauma to the middle or inner ear during the surgery (Guan et al. 2021).

9.2 Balance Function Assessment Methods

Interacting with input signals from the visual, vestibular, and proprioceptive systems results in normal motor function by establishing static and dynamic postures. There are three approaches to clinical balance assessment: functional assessment, system assessment, and quantitative assessment (Horak 1997). Posturography is the main quantitative and objective method for the evaluation of balance function, which analyzes the contribution of vestibular, visual, and proprioceptive inputs involved in maintaining an upright stance under static and dynamic conditions, respectively (Visser et al. 2008). Static posturography aims to measure postural sway in a subject who is standing as steady as possible, which is usually quantified by measuring the displacement of the center of pressure (Mancini and Horak 2010). In contrast, dynamic posturography uses experimentally induced balancing disturbances. When the support surface makes abrupt horizontal or vertical displacements, the balance might be disrupted. Slow and oscillatory perturbations have been used to study postural adaptation, stimulus anticipation, and feed-forward postural control mechanisms (Van Ooteghem et al. 2008), while quick and transient movements have been used to explore instantaneous defensive postural reactions and response latency. The performance of postural stability was not substantially altered by CI surgery.

9.2.1 Computerized Dynamic Posturography (CDP)

One of the most widely used quantitative methods for evaluating balance in humans is CDP, which includes sensory organization tests (SOT) and motor coordination assessment (Black 2001). SOT can be used to objectively measure postural stability. The participants completed all six of the SOT's conditions, including eyes open and closed, surrounding or platform fixed and swaying (Pletcher et al. 2017). Studies have assessed the impact of CI on postural control by comparing CDP scores, and the results showed that balance function improved significantly after implantation (Buchman et al. 2004). The improvement in balance function after CI could be explained by the fact that electrical stimulation might also provide input to the vestibular system. Meanwhile, some studies reported conflicting results, in which children after CI showed a significant increase in postural instability, which was more evident under dynamic conditions (Bayat et al. 2020). Compared with those without inner ear anomalies, the balance capability in patients with CI with inner ear anomalies was worse. More vestibular rehabilitation treatment plans are suggested for these patients (Hosseinzadeh et al. 2020).

9.3 Vestibular and Balance Function Pre- and Post-CI Surgery

Complaints of dizziness, vertigo, and imbalance are regularly reported post-CI surgery, so it has become increasingly crucial to examine vestibular function post-CI surgery (Piker et al. 2020). Two meta-analyses showed that the caloric test and cVEMP are the most commonly used vestibular function measurements in patients with CI (Abouzayd et al. 2017; Ibrahim et al. 2017). Due to its proximity to the cochlea, it is hypothesized that the saccule is the most susceptible to injury in vestibular end-organ following CI surgery; therefore, cVEMP will be affected. However, it should be noted that the cVEMP measurement is not standardized in the current clinic setting, e.g., the stimulus type varied among the literature, some utilized air-conducted tone bursts or clicks, and others used bone conduction. Furthermore, monitoring and rectification of electromyographic (EMG) activity of the sternocleidomastoid (SCM) muscle is essential for the precise recording of cVEMP (Rosengren et al. 2019), but not always adopted by the studies.

The caloric test is the most widely used vestibular function test in post-CI patients. However, CI surgery would potentially alter the temporal bone anatomy and, in turn, the heat transfer properties of the caloric test, making it difficult to determine whether the change in the results of the caloric test post-CI surgery reflects changes in vestibular function (Patki et al. 2016). Although the VOR test revealed reductions in response, it was not possible to identify patients who would experience vestibular symptoms after CI. CI could improve the patient's postural stability through mechanisms including vestibular compensation or electrical stimulation of the vestibular nerve or end organs (Buchman et al. 2004).

The vHIT has been used to quantify the function of horizontal and vertical semicircular canals. The vHIT test is a well-tolerated measurement that, unlike caloric testing, does not depend on heat transfer through the temporal bone. Studies indicated that vHIT was the least influenced vestibular test in CI surgery (Abouzayd et al. 2017). However, it should be noted that vHIT is associated only with the high-frequency range of vestibular function but not with daily activities (Halmagyi et al. 2017).

Both static and dynamic balance function tests could be used to assess post-CI patients. A study revealed that children with cochlear implants performed poorly on the dynamic balance function test compared to their counterparts with normal hearing, but showed minor improvements while the cochlear implants were switched on (Cushing et al. 2008). Another possible explanation for implant-induced improvement in balance function is due to electrical stimulation of the vestibular nerve, given the proximity of the cochlear and vestibular nerves and/or vestibular end organs. Many reports in the literature described discrete activation of the vestibular system, resulting in nystagmus and vertigo in patients with CI (Wong et al. 2000).

9.4 Vestibular Function of Patients with Cochlear Nerve Deficiency (CND)

Attention should be paid to vestibular nerve deficiency (VND), as well as vestibular dysfunction, in hearing loss patients with CND, although the rate of VND in patients with CND varied between studies, according to one of the latest studies, 14 of 38 patients (36.8%) showed hypoplasia or absence of vestibular nerve (Tsukada and Usami 2021). In a study evaluating pediatric sensorineural hearing loss with MRI, the authors reported that the absence of the vestibular nerve was observed in 13 of 49 ears (27%) with CND (McClay et al. 2008), and another study of the inner ear morphologic characteristics reported that a loss of the vestibular nerve was observed in 10 of 19 ears (53%) in CND cases (Adunka et al. 2006). Because the vestibular nerve is assumed to mature earlier than the cochlear nerve (Lim and Brichta 2016), vestibular nerve loss may always be accompanied by cochlear nerve deficiency; however, cochlear nerve deficiency is not always followed by vestibular nerve loss. Additionally, the hearing level showed worse results for those accompanied by VND in patients with CND.

Furthermore, the fact that 71% of patients with VND showed vestibular dysfunction, and 10 of 11 (90%) patients with vestibular dysfunction had VND suggests that vestibular dysfunction in patients with CND is partially due to the co-involvement of the vestibular nerve and cochlear hypoplasia (Tsukada and Usami 2021). MRI will help detect this kind of deformity.

The number of studies on the assessment of vestibular function in patients with CND is limited. In a study that analyzed 38 children with unilateral CND, 11 patients (29%) showed vestibular dysfunction on caloric tests or cVEMP or both, of which eight patients showed abnormal results on caloric and cVEMP tests, suggesting that both the superior and inferior vestibular nerve were involved in CND (Tsukada and Usami 2021). The cochlear nerve and superior vestibular nerves are often co-involved in the development of the eighth cranial nerve, but the cochlear nerve and inferior vestibular branch appear to be independent (Schuknecht et al. 1965). This was confirmed by a study that analyzed internal auditory meatus deformities in children (Ito et al. 2007); in five out of 10 patients with unilateral CND, the results of the caloric test were abnormal, with two absent and three with higher unilateral weakness. In contrast, normal VEMPs were recorded in nine ears, implying that the function of the inferior vestibular nerve is normal. Compared to the inferior branch, the risk of co-involvement of the cochlear nerve and superior vestibular nerve activities is higher.

Most patients with CND showed deterioration of vestibular function but were not completely absent, indicating that vestibular function persisted in most cases. According to a study by Tsukada and Usami, only two of the 11 patients with vestibular impairment were absent on the caloric test and cVEMP, while the remaining nine patients showed poor vestibular responses (Tsukada and Usami 2021). This revealed that the vestibular nerve and its function persist to some degree in most cases with VND, even if it cannot be detected by MRI.

Evaluating vestibular function will also help explain the discrepancy between the MRI-detected CND and auditory or speech outcomes after CI. Young et al. found open-set and closed-set speech perception in four children with CND (Young et al. 2012). One of the possible explanations is that some cochlear fibers travel alongside vestibular or even facial nerves, and anatomical studies have proven the existence of anastomotic connections between the branches of the cochlear and vestibular nerves (Tian et al. 2008; Kutz Jr et al. 2011; Vincenti et al. 2014). A normal result of the caloric and/or VEMP test will be useful to demonstrate the intact vestibular nerve.

Our center retrospectively analyzed preoperative vestibular function in 14 patients with CND, including 12 children and two adults, all of them completed the air-conducted cVEMP (AC-cVEMP) test before CI surgery. However, due to age limitation and cooperation ability, we performed caloric and vHIT tests only in two patients with CND before CI surgery. In the preoperative caloric test of the two patients with CND, no nystagmus was stimulated in either case under both conditions, showing deterioration of bilateral horizontal semicircular canal function.

Among them, 12 patients (85.71%) showed abnormal results in the cVEMP test, and two patients, including one child and one adult, had elicited a response to AC-cVEMP before CI, which showed typical P13 and N23 waveforms (Fig. 9.1). Nine patients participated in postoperative follow-up and completed the AC-cVEMP

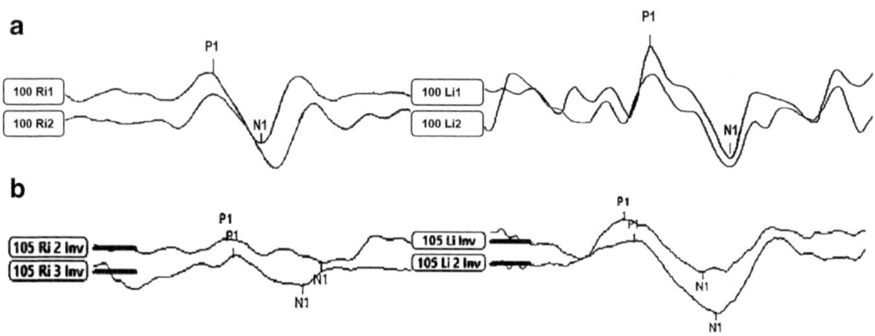

Fig. 9.1 (**a**) cVEMP results of the child with CND before surgery; (**b**) cVEMP results of the adult with CND before surgery. cVEMP, cervical vestibular evoked myogenic potential

test 1 month after CI surgery. However, no patients appeared with a cVEMP response in the implantation ear, including two patients who had a normal response before CI surgery.

The balance function in children with CND was acquired from their parents. Due to the age of the included children being <4 years old, we only evaluated their gross motor functions. In this cohort of 12 children with CND, the mean head control time was 4.25 months, and the mean independently walking time was 17.67 months. The results showed a significant delay in gross motor development of patients with CND compared to healthy children (head control at 3 months and independent walking at 12 months) (Bellman et al. 2013), which is similar to previous studies (Van Ooteghem et al. 2008; Kimura et al. 2018). Furthermore, patients with CND at our center had various inner ear malformations, and their delayed gross motor development and balance function may also be related to abnormal inner ear development (Kaga and Kimitaka 2017).

9.5 Conclusions

Various vestibular and balance function assessment methods could be used to evaluate patients with CND. The results of the caloric and VEMP tests are significantly influenced by CI surgery. CI surgery had a less significant effect on vHIT, posturography, or DHI scores. A substantial percentage of CND was also accompanied by a deficiency in the branches of the vestibular nerve, including the superior, inferior, or both. As a result, it is important to assess vestibular and balance functions in patients with CND pre- and post-CI surgery. There is a great discrepancy between vestibular or balance function performance and vertigo or dizziness symptoms in patients with CND pre- and post-CI surgery due to vestibular compensation from the central nervous system and potential stimulation of the vestibular nerve from the CI electrodes.

References

Abouzayd M, Smith PF, Moreau S, Hitier M. What vestibular tests to choose in symptomatic patients after a cochlear implant? A systematic review and meta-analysis. Eur Arch Otorhinolaryngol. 2017;274(1):53–63.

Adunka OF, Roush PA, Teagle HF, Brown CJ, Zdanski CJ, Jewells V, et al. Internal auditory canal morphology in children with cochlear nerve deficiency. Otol Neurotol. 2006;27(6):793–801.

Ajalloueyan M, Saeedi M, Sadeghi M, Abdollahi FZ. The effects of cochlear implantation on vestibular function in 1–4 years old children. Int J Pediatr Otorhinolaryngol. 2017;94:100–3.

Baloh RW, Sills AW, Honrubia V. Impulsive and sinusoidal rotatory testing: a comparison with results of caloric testing. Laryngoscope. 1979;89(4):646–54.

Bayat A, Farhadi M, Emamdjomeh H, Nadimi Z, Mirmomeni G. Influence of cochlear implantation on balance function in pediatrics. Int Tinnitus J. 2020;24(1):31–5.

Bellman M, Byrne O, Sege R. Developmental assessment of children [J]. BMJ. 2013;346:31–5.

Black FO. Clinical status of computerized dynamic posturography in neurotology. Curr Opin Otolaryngol Head Neck Surg. 2001;9(5):314–8.

Bogle J. The effect of Cochlear implantation on the vestibular evoked myogenic potential response in children and adults. Speech, Language, and Hearing Services Graduate Theses and Dissertations. 2010.

Buchman CA, Joy J, Hodges A, Telischi FF, Balkany TJ. Vestibular effects of cochlear implantation. Laryngoscope. 2004;114(10 Pt 2 Suppl 103):1–22. https://doi.org/10.1097/00005537-200410001-00001.

Colebatch J, Halmagyi G, Skuse N. Myogenic potentials generated by a click-evoked vestibulocollic reflex. J Neurol Neurosurg Psychiatry. 1994;57(2):190–7.

Cushing SL, Chia R, James AL, Papsin BC, Gordon KA. A test of static and dynamic balance function in children with cochlear implants: the vestibular olympics. Arch Otolaryngol Head Neck Surg. 2008;134(1):34–8. https://doi.org/10.1001/archoto.2007.16.

Dyde RT, Jenkin MR, Harris LR. The subjective visual vertical and the perceptual upright. Exp Brain Res. 2006;173(4):612–22.

Guan R, Wang Y, Wu S, Zhang B, Sun J, Guo X, et al. Vestibular function in children and adults before and after unilateral or sequential bilateral Cochlear implantation. Front Neurol. 2021;12:675502.

Halmagyi G, Aw S, Cremer P, Curthoys I, Todd M. Impulsive testing of individual semicircular canal function. Ann N Y Acad Sci. 2001;942(1):192–200.

Halmagyi GM, Chen L, MacDougall HG, Weber KP, McGarvie LA, Curthoys IS. The video head impulse test. Front Neurol. 2017;8 https://doi.org/10.3389/fneur.2017.00258.

Horak FB. Clinical assessment of balance disorders. Gait Posture. 1997;6(1):76–84.

Hosseinzadeh F, Asghari A, Moradi-Lakeh M, Farhadi M, Daneshi A, Mohseni M, et al. Balance function after cochlear implant and inner ear anomaly: comparison of dynamic posturography. Laryngoscope Investigative Otolaryngology. 2020;5(3):529–35.

Ibrahim I, da Silva SD, Segal B, Zeitouni A. Effect of cochlear implant surgery on vestibular function: meta-analysis study. Journal of Otolaryngology-Head & Neck Surgery. 2017;46(1):1–10.

Ito K, Ishimoto S-I, Karino S. Isolated cochlear nerve hypoplasia with various internal auditory meatus deformities in children. Annals of Otology, Rhinology & Laryngology. 2007;116(7):520–4.

Jacobson GP, Newman CW. The development of the dizziness handicap inventory. Archives of Otolaryngology–Head & Neck Surgery. 1990;116(4):424–7.

Jacot E, Van Den Abbeele T, Debre HR, Wiener-Vacher SR. Vestibular impairments pre-and post-cochlear implant in children. Int J Pediatr Otorhinolaryngol. 2009;73(2):209–17.

Kaga and Kimitaka. Cochlear implantation in children with inner ear malformation and cochlear nerve deficiency. Singapore: Springer; 2017.

Kimura Y, Masuda T, et al. Vestibular function and gross motor development in 195 children with congenital hearing loss-assessment of inner ear malformations. Otol Neurotol. 2018;39(2):196–205.

Kutz JW Jr, Lee KH, Isaacson B, Booth TN, Sweeney MH, Roland PS. Cochlear implantation in children with cochlear nerve absence or deficiency. Otol Neurotol. 2011;32(6):956–61.

Lim R, Brichta AM. Anatomical and physiological development of the human inner ear. Hear Res. 2016;338:9–21.

Mancini M, Horak FB. The relevance of clinical balance assessment tools to differentiate balance deficits. Eur J Phys Rehabil Med. 2010;46(2):239–48.

McClay JE, Booth TN, Parry DA, Johnson R, Roland P. Evaluation of pediatric sensorineural hearing loss with magnetic resonance imaging. Archives of Otolaryngology–Head & Neck Surgery. 2008;134(9):945–52.

Melvin T-AN, Della Santina CC, Carey JP, Migliaccio AA. The effects of cochlear implantation on vestibular function. Otology & neurotology: official publication of the American Otological Society, American Neurotology Society [and] European academy of Otology and Neurotology. 2009;30(1):87.

Patki AU, Ronen O, Kaylie DM, Frank-Ito DO, Piker EG. Anatomic variations in temporal bones affect the intensity of nystagmus during warm caloric irrigation. Otol Neurotol. 2016;37(8):1111–6. https://doi.org/10.1097/mao.0000000000001129.

Pavlou M, Whitney S, Alkathiry AA, Huett M, Luxon LM, Raglan E, et al. The pediatric vestibular symptom questionnaire: a validation study. J Pediatr. 2016;168:171–7.

Piker EG, Riska K, Garrison D, Kaylie DM. Vestibular function after cochlear implantation: a test battery and case-by-case approach. Laryngoscope Investig Otolaryngol. 2020;5(3):560–71. https://doi.org/10.1002/lio2.413.

Pletcher ER, Williams VJ, Abt JP, Morgan PM, Parr JJ, Wohleber MF, et al. Normative data for the NeuroCom sensory organization test in US military special operations forces. J Athl Train. 2017;52(2):129–36. https://doi.org/10.4085/1062-6050-52.1.05.

Psillas G, Pavlidou A, Lefkidis N, Vital I, Markou K, Triaridis S, et al. Vestibular evoked myogenic potentials in children after cochlear implantation. Auris Nasus Larynx. 2014;41(5):432–5.

Rosengren S, Todd NM, Colebatch J. Vestibular-evoked extraocular potentials produced by stimulation with bone-conducted sound. Clin Neurophysiol. 2005;116(8):1938–48.

Rosengren SM, Colebatch JG, Young AS, Govender S, Welgampola MS. Vestibular evoked myogenic potentials in practice: methods, pitfalls and clinical applications. Clin Neurophysiol Pract. 2019;4:47–68.

Schuknecht HF, Icarashi M, Gacek RR. The pathological types of cochleo-saccular degeneration. Acta Otolaryngol. 1965;59(2–6):154–70.

Shepard N, Jacobson G. The caloric irrigation test. Handb Clin Neurol. 2016;137:119–31.

Tian G-Y, Xu D-C, Huang D-L, Liao H, Huang M-X. The topographical relationships and anastomosis of the nerves in the human internal auditory canal. Surg Radiol Anat. 2008;30(3):243–7. https://doi.org/10.1007/s00276-008-0311-z.

Tsukada K, Usami S-I. Vestibular nerve deficiency and vestibular function in children with unilateral hearing loss caused by cochlear nerve deficiency. Acta Otolaryngol. 2021;141(9):835–40.

Van Ooteghem K, Frank J, Allard F, Buchanan J, Oates A, Horak F. Compensatory postural adaptations during continuous, variable amplitude perturbations reveal generalized rather than sequence-specific learning. Exp Brain Res. 2008;187(4):603–11.

Vincenti V, Ormitti F, Ventura E, Guida M, Piccinini A, Pasanisi E. Cochlear implantation in children with cochlear nerve deficiency. Int J Pediatr Otorhinolaryngol. 2014;78(6):912–7. https://doi.org/10.1016/j.ijporl.2014.03.003.

Visser JE, Carpenter MG, van der Kooij H, Bloem BR. The clinical utility of posturography. Clin Neurophysiol. 2008;119(11):2424–36. https://doi.org/10.1016/j.clinph.2008.07.220.

Wong EC, See HK, Yu HC. The phenomenon of nystagmus upon electrical stimulation in a cochlear implant patient. Adv Otorhinolaryngol. 2000;57:189–91. https://doi.org/10.1159/000059233.

Young NM, Kim FM, Ryan ME, Tournis E, Yaras S. Pediatric cochlear implantation of children with eighth nerve deficiency. Int J Pediatr Otorhinolaryngol. 2012;76(10):1442–8. https://doi.org/10.1016/j.ijporl.2012.06.019.

Diagnosis and Treatment Strategies for Cochlear Nerve Deficiency: A Summary of the Entire Book

Yongxin Li

Based on all the chapters' content, we summed up a flow diagram of diagnosis and treatment strategies for cochlear nerve deficiency (CND) which may be caused by embryonic development problem or acquired degeneration such as cytomegalovirus infection (Fig. A1). The diagnosis of CND is operated by magnetic resonance

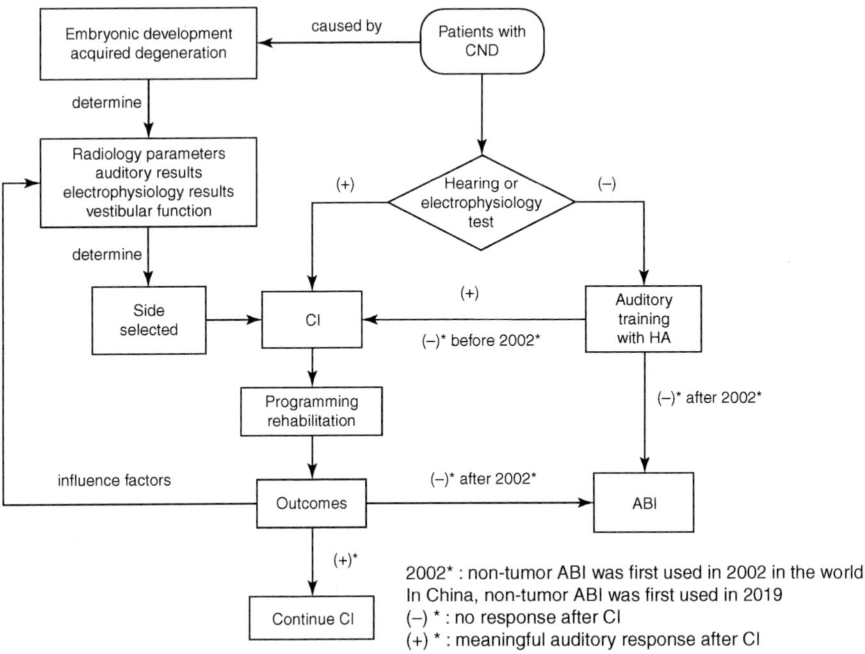

Fig. A1 The flow diagram of diagnosis and treatment strategies for cochlear nerve deficiency patients

Y. Li (ed.), *Cochlear Implantation for Cochlear Nerve Deficiency*,
https://doi.org/10.1007/978-981-19-5892-2

imaging (MRI) as both computerized tomography (CT) and MRI parameters of CND have their own specificity. The auditory and electrophysiology test results of CND patients are usually insufficient. When a CND patient has residual hearing, we can do cochlear implantation (CI) for the patient to obtain hearing. However, when a CND patient has no residual hearing, we can do auditory training with powerful hearing aid for the patient, if auditory response can be elicited and CI can be perfumed. Before 2002, when auditory brainstem implant (ABI) was first applied to non-tumor cases, even the CND patient after auditory training had no auditory response, and at that time, when the patients or their families urged CI, we could try CI for them. After 2002, ABI was applied for CND patients who had no auditory response. The CI side selected strategy was based on radiology parameters (nerve bundles in the internal auditory canal, diameter of bony cochlear nerve canal, inner ear malformation, and so on), auditory and electrophysiology results, and so on. Recently, vestibular function has been also considered as a determined factor. The detailed selected strategies of CI for CND patients have been discussed at the fore. The CI outcomes were also affected by radiology parameters, auditory results, and so on. If the patient had no response after CI, ABI could be performed. If there were meaningful auditory response after CI, the patients could continue using CI, and regular programming and rehabilitation should be performed for better results.

Printed by Printforce, the Netherlands